D0872808

ACUTE HEAD INJURY

FORTHCOMING TITLES

Occupational Therapy for the Brain-Injured Adult
Jo Clark-Wilson and Gordon Muir Giles

Multiple Sclerosis
Approaches to management
Lorraine De Souza

Modern Electrotherapy
Mary Dyson and Christopher Hayne

Autism
A multidisciplinary approach
Edited by Kathryn Ellis

Physiotherapy in Respiratory and Intensive Care
Alexandra Hough

Community Occupational Therapy with Mentally Handicapped People
Debbie Isaac

Understanding Dysphasia
Lesley Jordan and Rita Twiston Davies

Management in Occupational Therapy
Zielfa B. Maslin

Keyboard, Graphic and Handwriting Skills
Helping people with motor disabilities
Dorothy E. Penso

Dysarthria
Theory and therapy
Sandra J. Robertson

Speech and Language Problems in Children
Dilys A. Treharne

THERAPY IN PRACTICE SERIES

Edited by Jo Campling

This series of books is aimed at 'therapists' concerned with rehabilitation in a very broad sense. The intended audience particularly includes occupational therapists, physiotherapists and speech therapists, but many titles will also be of interest to nurses, psychologists, medical staff, social workers, teachers or volunteer workers. Some volumes will be interdisciplinary, others aimed at one particular profession. All titles will be comprehensive but concise, and practical but with due reference to relevant theory and evidence. They are not research monographs but focus on professional practice, and will be of value to both students and qualified personnel.

Acute Head Injury

Practical management in rehabilitation

RUTH GARNER

Therapy in Practice 13

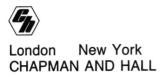

London   New York
CHAPMAN AND HALL

First published in 1990 by
Chapman and Hall Ltd
11 New Fetter Lane, London EC4P 4EE

Published in the USA by
Chapman and Hall
29 West 35th Street, New York NY10001

© 1990 Ruth Garner

Typeset in 10/12 Times by
Mayhew Typesetting, Bristol
Printed in Great Britain by
St. Edmundsbury Press, Bury St. Edmunds, Suffolk

ISBN 0 412 32420 2

British Library Cataloguing in Publication Data

Garner, Ruth
   Acute head injury: Practical management in
   rehabilitation. – (Therapy in practice; 13).
   1. Head injured patients. Rehabilitation
   I. Title II. Series
   362.1'9751

   ISBN 0 412 32420 2

Library of Congress Cataloging in Publication Data
available.

To my mother and father,
Ruth and Bill Thomas,
and to my husband Frank

Contents

Acknowledgements

My many thanks go to those who have provided help and guidance by reading and commenting on parts of this book; these include Karen Jones, Liz Wakely, Wyn Jones-Owen, Jackie Berisford and Rosemary Jenkins. Thanks also go to other colleagues at the Birmingham Accident Hospital, who have been supportive over the years, and with whom it has been a pleasure to work. Without the support of staff within the Occupational Therapy Department and the help and encouragement of Marianne Colbear, District Occupational Therapist, the task of writing a book would have been a far more arduous one.

I am indebted to the members of Headway West Midlands for allowing me to be part of this organization. I am particularly grateful to Karen Oakly for giving me permission to include a part of her private diary to illustrate the text and to Marion Hemmings for sharing her experiences with me. There are too many dedicated members to mention by name, but I have always considered the work of this group to be invaluable in the support they provide both for families and members of the caring profession.

My special thanks go to Mr P.S. London, currently Honorary Consulting Surgeon at the Birmingham Accident Hospital, who has given me considerable encouragement and guidance during the preparation of this manuscript, as well as during my career. Mr London, over many years, has made a significant contribution to the treatment of head-injured victims and was one of the first to acknowledge the burden that such patients place on the family and community at the time of discharge from hospital. I am proud and privileged to have worked with him.

Finally, thanks go to my husband, Frank, for being so patient during long periods of my preoccupation with the word-processor, for providing a proof-reading service and for having faith.

Foreword

It is both a pleasure and a privilege to be invited to contribute a foreword to this book, which deserves – and needs – to be read by virtually everyone who is concerned with the treatment and subsequent welfare of the victims of severe injuries of the brain. Some friends, relatives and workmates might be helped by reading some parts of it, but, if the book has the effect it deserves to have on therapists, nurses, doctors, and others working in both hospitals and the community, these laymen will be suitably informed and assisted by one or more members of the necessarily large therapeutic team.

The improvements in methods of resuscitation that have taken place during the last 40 years or so have abolished the previously fatalistic readiness to accept that a week or two in coma after a head injury was virtually a sentence to death from pneumonia. After it had become possible to save lives it gradually became clear that survival of the patient was not necessarily followed by recovery of the brain and that the price of success, in saving lives, was a population of cerebral cripples that was increasing at the rate of 1000 or more a year throughout the country. Although this figure has remained about the same for more than 20 years, there has been a great improvement in the amount of interest, the standard of care and the quality of results that are being achieved. The explanation of this apparent contradiction is most probably that the less severely injured are making better recoveries and the more severely injured are surviving. In other words, today's handicapped survivors come from a more severely injured group than did the survivors of a generation ago.

The remarkable improvements in treatment and results originated in a small, but devoted, group of pioneers under the leadership of Mr P.P. Lockhart, Head Almoner; Miss A. Savage, Head Occupational Therapist; Mr J.V. Thackeray, Head Remedial Gymnast; and Mr H. Proctor, a surgeon at the Birmingham Accident Hospital; rehabilitation units of the Royal Air Force worked with them. Their methods were based on recognizing that it is as necessary to stimulate an injured brain in order to help it to recover as it is to stimulate a normal brain to enable it to develop – a process that has rather nicely been referred to as 'exercising the mental muscles'.

Mrs Garner was an early and enthusiastic recruit to this therapeutic team, in which, and beyond which, she advanced to a position of leadership; that is no small achievement when one considers the size and complexity of the team that has spread from hospitals to homes, schools and places of work. She has now made available the results of her and her colleagues' work in Birmingham in an essentially practical guide to the care of the victims of severe injuries of the brain, paying particular attention to the disturbances of behaviour, which are so much more difficult to deal with than the purely physical disabilities.

This book will be of particular value to occupational and physiotherapists, but speech therapists, psychologists and social workers will find much here to add to their understanding of the wider implications of severe injuries of the brain. Because therapists need to start treating patients while they are still receiving intensive care, nurses in these units, as well as those in ordinary wards, need to know how closely their work should be integrated with that of others. Doctors who read this book may not find much of the practical detail relevant to their role, but they will derive great benefit from such clear evidence of the range and duration of methods of treatment required and of the fact that they have a part to play long after the patients leave hospital.

P.S. London, MBE, FRCS, MFOM
Honorary Consulting Surgeon
to the Birmingham Accident Hospital

1

Introduction

Over the past few years there has been an increase in the number of patients surviving head injury and with this has come a greater understanding of the nature and extent of the problem, although much is yet to be researched. Within the general hospital we are likely to encounter survivors of head injury, mild, moderate and severe, and so we should have the knowledge to deal with the initial problems and prevent further complications. In this we all have a significant contribution to make.

This guide to practice hopes to cover aspects of head-injury rehabilitation from the time of admission to the time of discharge from inpatient care. In the absence of appropriate resources in this country, the period of time in attending a hospital for treatment, as opposed to attending a suitable rehabilitation centre, may be extended beyond that which one might desire. Alternatively, due to lack of resources and lack of knowledge, many head-injured patients are discharged too early, with hospital personnel failing to realize the burden this places on the family who are left to cope as best they can.

The early treatment of the head-injured patient excludes no-one; therefore this guide is aimed at all disciplines who may come into contact with such patients or their families. Early treatment concentrates on sensory stimulation, facilitation of function, prevention of complications and return to the community. However, the patients' problems do not end at discharge, but, in many instances, only just begin. Attention, therefore, should finally be focused on the psychosocial consequences of head injury which recognize that the primary long-term problems encountered are generally not of a physical nature.

The text generally relates to adult patients, although children may be mentioned, particularly in relation to the sensory stimulation programme. It is important that children, with developing rather than developed minds, are seen as being in need of paediatricians' care and early referral to an appropriate unit is essential.

THE EXTENT OF THE PROBLEM

A report by the Medical Disability Society's working party (1987), estimated that the annual incidence of severe head injury is approximately eight per 100 000 population in the United Kingdom, with two of these, six months after injury, still being in the stage of severe disability or coma. Moderate head injury is estimated to be at a rate of approximately 18 per 100 000 population per annum. In each health district (averaging a population of 250 000), it is estimated that the number of disabled survivors at any one time will amount to between 250 and 375, exacerbated by the prolonged duration of recovery and long life expectancy.

Head injury occurs commonly in young males between the ages of 17 and 22 years who may have many years to live, in many cases presenting problems of long-term rehabilitation and/or care. This needs to be considered when setting long-term goals, as, if the patient returns to live with parents, the life expectancy of the patient could easily exceed that of the carers.

CLASSIFICATION OF HEAD INJURY

Traumatic brain injury, as defined by the Medical Disability Society (1987), is 'Brain injury caused by trauma to the head (including the effects upon the brain of other possible complications of injury, notably hypoxaemia and hypotension, and intracerebral haematoma).'

Closed-head injury is the result of acceleration or deceleration impact of the brain within the confines of the skull and results in diffuse damage. There is localized damage at the site of impact, and, in many instances, of the opposite pole as well (Contrecoup). There is accompanying diffuse shearing of axons due to the rotary motion of the brain. This primary damage is a result of mechanical factors and is seldom affected by treatment. Secondary complications commonly occur and result in further damage and may include intracranial haematoma, cerebral oedema and infection.

Glasgow Coma Scale

'Coma is defined as "no eye opening, no uttering of words, no obedience to commands", no matter how strong a stimulation is applied' (Jennett *et al.*, 1976). The Glasgow Coma Scale (GCS) is a method frequently used to categorize the levels of responsiveness following head injury, and, as depth and duration of coma are recognized as reliable indicators of possible outcome, this information is valuable in long-term planning. The GCS involves recording eye opening, best verbal response and best motor response, assigning a score to each and then adding them (most responsive being a total of 15 and least responsive being three). This is an easily applied and reliable measure (Jennett *et al.*, 1979).

Severe head injury is defined as a score of eight or less for a minimum of six hours. A moderate head injury is a score of between nine and 11, and a mild injury is a score of 12 or more.

Post-traumatic amnesia

Post-traumatic amnesia (PTA) also relates well to outcome and is defined as the time between injury and return to full consciousness. The advantage of PTA is that the severity of injury can be assessed in conversation with the patient months after injury and without reference to the patient's records.

PTA for less than one hour characterizes a mild injury, for between one and 24 hours a moderate injury, for between one and seven days a severe injury and for more than seven days a very severe injury (Russell, 1932).

Caution should be practised in the estimation of full consciousness, as this entails the return of full memory and not spasmodic memory of events.

COURSE OF RECOVERY

The course of recovery will be dependent on the severity of injury, as well as on the complications experienced.

3

Mild head injury

Those with a GCS of 12 or more following injury, with PTA for less than 60 minutes, may return to normal activity within a few days following injury but may experience dizziness, impaired concentration, fatigue, depression, irritability, headaches and memory disorder for up to, and sometimes beyond, three months. These symptoms may affect performance at work, although this may be subtle.

Moderate head injury

Those with a GCS of nine to 11, or PTA of between one and 24 hours, may exhibit disorders of a physical, cognitive and behavioural nature, in varying degrees and combinations. Following a moderate injury, intensive rehabilitation is required for up to, and often in excess of, 12 months. Return to employment may be achievable.

Severe head injury

Those with a GCS of less than eight will exhibit disorders of a physical, cognitive and behavioural nature of varying degrees and combinations. Prolonged rehabilitation is required, and if independence is regained it may take years. Return to work may not be possible and attendance at a sheltered workshop may be more appropriate for many patients.

Outcome

Jennett and Bond (1975) have classified outcome as:

1. No recovery from coma until death.
2. Vegetative state: breathing spontaneously, spontaneous eye opening, reflex responses to deep pain and swallowing of food placed in the mouth may be seen.
3. Severe disability: conscious but requires help in some activities of daily living. Dependence is due to a combination of physical and mental disabilities.
4. Moderate disability: independent but disabled.

5. Good recovery: indicates capacity to resume normal work and social activity, although for various reasons the former may not happen.

PROGNOSTIC CONSIDERATIONS

Reports in the literature refer to recovery periods ranging from six months to decades following injury, with average periods in hospital from three to six months. LeMay and Geschwind (1978) found that the maximum recovery following closed head injury in children under five years of age might take decades; people aged 20 to 40 years continued to improve for up to five years; people of 40 to 60 years improve for up to two years following injury; and those beyond the age of 60 ceased to improve within nine months.

Groher (1977) and Gruzzman (1982) suggested that the greatest degree of recovery occurs within the first six months of injury, with slow progress being made after this. Within the first six months, they suggest that the greatest degree of recovery takes place within the first month.

Premorbid personality and behaviour appear to have a significant influence on recovery. Individuals who are strong-willed, self-motivated and driven to accomplish positive goals with good track-records at school and at work, tend to do better than those with emotional and psychological instability, a history of alcohol or drug abuse, poor work and/or school record and general lack of motivation to accomplish positive goals (Adamovitch et al., 1985).

Greater recovery appears to be seen when families and others concerned are supportive and involved in the rehabilitation process. This is an important consideration for health-service workers, who must ensure that families are encouraged to become constructively involved in the care of the head-injured relative and are educated in the rehabilitation process early on.

CLINICAL FEATURES

Each severely head-injured patient is unique in the complexity of the clinical picture he may present to the treatment team, and rehabilitation can be a daunting challenge.

The physical disorders which may be presented include altered tone in one or any combination of the four limbs, altered sensation, abnormal reflexes and posture, poor co-ordination, and a restricted range of movement. These may be accompanied by other injuries sustained at the time of injury including fractures, lacerations and skin loss, burns and internal injuries, for example of liver, bowel and spleen.

The patient will experience altered perception, particularly during the initial phase of recovery and this may be in any combination of seeing, hearing, feeling, tasting and smelling. As the patient becomes more aware many of these disorders will abate.

Cognitive disorders following head injury may include lack of insight, disorientation, reduced attention, impaired memory and decreased ability in the processing of information. These will become more apparent with an increase in the patient's level of awareness. Cognitive disorders have significant implications for rehabilitation.

Behavioural disorders may be transitory or prolonged. These may include verbal or physical aggression, apathy, agitation, distractability and inappropriate use of social skills. A personality change will often accompany head injury and minor traits seen within the previous personality may be heightened.

THE TREATMENT TEAM

An integrated interdisciplinary team is essential in the treatment of the head-injured patient. It is inappropriate for disciplines to work in isolation, as they may individually strive to collect the same information and base-line measurements, may confuse the patient by adopting differing treatment strategies, may present conflicting information to relatives, may assume that important areas of assessment and treatment are being dealt with by others, and, in short, fail to provide an effective and efficient co-ordinated rehabilitation programme.

The doctor, in the UK, leads the treatment team and should have an interest in the treatment of the patient over and above that of the medical management, and should recognize the contribution that the other disciplines have to make to the rehabilitation of such patients. An experienced consultant, with a commitment to the rehabilitation of the head-injured patient, provides a firm foundation from which the treatment team can operate. We must not forget that the doctor is legally responsible for the clinical care of the patient, for the allocation of beds, and referral of the patient to, or for, other services.

The nurses provide 24-hour care for the patient and are important team members by the very nature of providing a consistent treatment approach. Rehabilitation does not only take place during the working day, but requires reinforcing during the evenings and weekends. Nurses are always available to talk to relatives, and in so doing, are able to offer support. During the period of coma, nurses are able to play a valuable part in providing the stimulation that is essential for the recovery of the brain.

The physiotherapist plays an important role in the prevention of deformity and in the facilitation of normal movement. This team member must be instrumental in advising other team members, including relatives, in appropriate techniques of positioning and in transferring the patient from one position to another. The physiotherapist has other vital roles to play, such as in maintaining clear airways.

The occupational therapist is a versatile team member who has skills to offer both in cognitive assessment and treatment, as well as in retraining of functional skills. He/she has a valuable part to play from the stage of sensory stimulation to independence in the community, being the one to assess for disability equipment and adaptation to the home and being the one to initiate early home visits. If unable to transfer the patient to suitable rehabilitation facilities, he/she is able to assess and retrain in work-associated activities. The occupational therapist recognizes the importance of independence in leisure activities.

The psychologist is essential for guidance in early management of behavioural problems, as well as in the assessment of cognitive functions. Advice should be sought from psychologists by all team members about measures which may be adopted in order to improve the effectiveness of treatment.

The speech therapist should be introduced to the patient early in his treatment in order to assess and provide advice on the management of disorders of swallowing and language. Speech therapists are generally limited in the time they are able to give to individual patients, and after assessment will often provide exercises which other team members can execute.

The social worker has a part to play in the assistance given to families dealing with financial problems resulting from the injury, and other practical issues such as providing help with other dependants. The support of the social worker, often perceived as being apart from the other team members, is invaluable throughout the period of hospitalization and in the return to the community, both to the family members and later to the patient himself.

Each hospital will have differing strengths within each discipline according to resources, expertise, experience, interest and individual personalities.

The key worker

It is advisable, in many instances, to identify a key worker for each patient who will co-ordinate the individual rehabilitation programme and communicate information to the family and other team members. This key worker should be identified as the patient's level of awareness improves and may be chosen either because of the significant role she/he plays in the rehabilitation programme, in accordance with the specific needs of the patient, or because of the positive relationship which may have been formed either between him/herself and the patient or family. The key worker may be changed as the patient progresses and a community key worker may need to be identified early in order to provide continuity of care after discharge from hospital.

REHABILITATION DEFINED

Rehabilitation has been described in a steering committee report (A Rehabilitation Service for the West Midlands, 1987), as 'a process intended to enable disabled persons to play as active, independent and satisfying a part in everyday life as possible. For some this means the medical and other care that enables them to resume all their previous activities after temporary disablement by illness or injury. For others, disablement continues though it may improve or fluctuate about a steady level.'

2

Early intervention

Even in the earliest stages after admission to hospital there is much
that can be done by all members of the treatment team to provide
the severely head-injured patient with an environment that is
conducive to promoting the recovery of the nervous system and so
the patient as a whole.

There is evidence that initiating a rehabilitation programme early
after onset of head injury helps to reduce the long-term effects, and,
in doing so, shorten the total period of rehabilitation. Cope and Hall
(1982) conducted a four-year study at the Santa Clara Valley
Medical Centre, and found that intervention within 35 days of injury
led to an earlier discharge than for those whose rehabilitation
programme began later than 35 days after injury.

Factors which were considered to be responsible for the beneficial
effects of an early start to rehabilitation included: ultimate potential
recovery could be realized (relating plasticity to interval of time after
injury), avoidance of medical complications, control of the environment enabling channelling of meaningful stimulation, adoption of a
routine, prevention of behavioural problems, and the involvement of
the family who were educated in the rehabilitation process.

AIMS OF TREATMENT

1. For those patients in the primary stage, the aim is to raise the
   level of awareness by using controlled stimulation of all five
   senses.
2. To use the position of the patient to prevent/correct physical disability, providing him with the best position in which to experience,
   and interact with, the stimulations provided by the environment.

9

3. To educate, and involve, the family in the rehabilitation process and, in doing so, provide support.

KNOWING THE PATIENT

It is most important to know as much about the patient before setting overall aims and planning treatment. Important sources of information include:

1. The relatives, or close friends.
2. If the patient is a child, the school, college or university which can be approached by the hospital teacher, if one exists.
3. Workmates.
4. The hospital social work department, if they have become involved, or the local social services department.

The interview with the relatives

The term 'relatives' is intended to include anyone with a close personal relationship with the patient. Ideally, this will take place before the evaluation period but this may not be the best time for obtaining all the information required. Repeated interviews should be arranged as necessary to discuss developments, as well as seek new information. The interview is for the purpose of:

1. Getting to know about the patient as a person.
2. Providing an explanation, in simple terms, of the purpose of rehabilitation.
3. Requesting familiar objects, for example records and photographs, to be brought in for the patient, and used during treatment sessions.
4. Providing support for the relatives.
5. Building a rapport with the family.

The Personal History Sheet (see Figure 2.1) should cover family background, including siblings' names and ages, type of relationships existing, nicknames, and so on. It includes the name of the school, college, or current employer and the name of a personal teacher or an immediate supervisor at work. Details of work history are important, as are qualifications gained. Information about patients' educational attainments are always helpful.

Figure 2.1: The Personal History Sheet used by the Occupational Therapy Department at the Birmingham Accident Hospital and Rehabilitation Centre.

Personal history sheet

Name: Hosp. Num: Age:

Diagnosis: Team: Date:

Home address:

Next of kin:

Siblings:

School and teacher's name:

Employment:

Employer's name:

Educational attainments:

Names of friends:

Hobbies and general interests:

Personality and character:

General information:

History given by

Relationship to patient

It is useful to know the names of the patient's friends (familiar names) and their particular relationship to the patient. Relatives should be asked about the patients' personality but the information they give is generally inaccurate at this point. As the rapport grows, relatives will be able to give more information with greater accuracy. Sometimes friends are more informative than relatives, which can lead to difficulties if they are not on good terms with the family.

Hobbies and interests are a useful basis for treatment sessions. What does the patient do in his spare time? Where does he go in the evenings or at weekends? What type of programmes does he watch/listen to on the television and radio? What type of newspaper/magazine does he read? His likes and dislikes should be

11

known, particularly in eating and drinking – does he take milk and sugar in coffee? The medical history may have covered any previous disability, but it is worth checking whether the patient wears glasses, has a hearing-aid, and whether he has any physical deformities, habits or obsessions. Any previous psychiatric history is particularly relevant.

To accompany the personal history, the relatives should be asked to bring a selection of familiar objects which the patient previously found comforting to the hospital, for example tapes of favourite music, and large, good-quality photographs clearly labelled on the back. The photographs need to be of an individual person, animal or object, which has meaning for the patient. These items are useful in treatment sessions only if one is aware of the relationship to the patient, and, therefore, can associate activities with these objects in a meaningful way.

EVALUATION

It is necessary to understand the patient's condition in detail in order to establish a base-line for treatment. As with any early treatment sessions, the environment in which evaluation is conducted should be one in which stimulation can be channelled, and in which the patient is given the opportunity to attend to the therapist without distraction. Unfortunately, in many busy hospitals such a place is often difficult to find.

Evaluation must be both through observation of, and interaction with, the patient. Careful notes should be taken to record all the responses, that is, stimulation given, time taken to respond, duration of response, quality and consistency. It is recommended that two people are present at the evaluation: one to work with the patient and one to record the responses, for it is easy to overlook these. It is also of value if those present have different professional backgrounds, and, therefore, different skills.

Initially the sessions should not last longer than 10 to 15 minutes, but these can be conducted about three times a day, depending on the tolerance of the patient. The timing of a session needs thought so that it will not directly follow another procedure which has tired the patient, for example a nursing process or a visit from a relative.

To prepare for the evaluation it is necessary to study the patient's medical history. Information required includes the patient's age, time between injury and evaluation, duration of coma (if applicable), and GCS rating.

The type of injury and the site will have implications for the prognosis, and additional injuries sustained will have implications for planning treatment. Medication needs to be noted and the effects of this taken into consideration during evaluation and treatment. Any previous medical history relevant to outcome should also be noted.

Evaluation of the patient should include position and posture, motor skills, sensorimotor function, eye movements and head and body control (Walstrom, 1983; Zoltan and Meeder Rykman, 1985).

Physical evaluation

The initial physical evaluation should be by observing the patient, but not when he is receiving attention from anyone or reacting with other people.

The areas to be evaluated include the range and quality of movement; whether or not movement is voluntary or spontaneous; whether responses are imitative or to command; and whether they are localized, generalized or reflexive. When testing for tone one should estimate the degree of flaccidity or spasticity and note contractures.

Decorticate or decerebrate spasticity or rigidity may result in contractures of muscle and soft tissue. Decerebrate rigidity also restricts movements of respiration. Decorticate posture is one of adduction of the shoulders, severe flexion of the elbows and wrists, and hyperextension of the joints of the lower limbs. In decerebrate posture there is extension of both upper and lower limbs. After head injury, these postures may be mixed or may alternate from one to the other in the same patient.

The patient's ability to sit, balance, and control his head should be assessed. Great caution should be exercised in this if the patient has not previously been placed in an upright position; the patient's respiration and heart-rate should be monitored throughout.

Responses to deliberate stimulation

This evaluation should involve responses to sound, touch, and smell; and responses should be recorded as delayed or absent, together with duration, and whether general or local, voluntary or reflex, appropriate or inappropriate, and away from or towards stimuli. The quality of the responses should also be noted.

No special equipment is necessary during evaluation but a little thought and imagination are required to make use of what is commonly available to the therapist. When testing reactions, use extremes of stimuli: hard and soft, hot and cold, loud and quiet, and pleasant and unpleasant odours, using both the familiar and the unfamiliar.

Sounds

Observe the patient when a member of staff is talking to him or when a close relative is speaking. How does he respond when you make a sudden noise, as when banging a drum, or make a familiar sound, as when clapping your hands or jingling keys, or when you play some familiar music.

Touch

Deep pain is tested by pinching the ear-lobes and other parts of the body, or by putting pressure on the nail beds with a hard object. Observe the patient during general touch, when applying different textures, and during rubbing of a part of the body.

Smell

Record the patient's responses to noxious odours which are believed to have an arousing effect, and to pleasant odours which are believed to have a calming effect.

Visual skills

During the assessment of eye movements, the patient, wherever possible, should be in an upright position. The first point to note is whether the patient opens his eyes, or can be encouraged to do so by gentle upward stroking of the lids, followed by holding the lids open for a short while.

If the patient is able to open his eyes, note how he attends to an interesting object or to yourself. How long does it take the patient to react? Note the quality of his response. The author generally uses a bright, coloured, familiar object belonging to the patient, or a mirror if there are no facial injuries or if the features are not changed. If the patient can attend to an object, can he follow it from side to side and up and down? If he can, what are his movements like: are they delayed, jerky, or smooth? Watch the patient in other circumstances, such as when a relative is moving around.

At a higher level, if the patient is able to respond to simple commands, can he point to a named colour when two colours are presented, or can he point to a named shape when two shapes are presented to him?

Communication

It is essential early on to find what means of communication can be used. At the lowest level, this may be by using a simple movement such as closing the eye, moving a hand, or pointing, or by the use of a sound. All who look after the patient, including the relatives, should know what means of communication is to be used and then should be consistent in its use.

Such simple means of communication are, one hopes, only temporary, but they are useful for offering the patient some control over his environment, allowing him to make some of his needs known; it can also be a means of showing his potential for recovery by demonstrating his level of awareness.

Summary of evaluation

Therapists and relatives alike should be aware that a patient's response must be consistent before it can be accepted as a response to a given stimulus. For example many patients have been reported to have said a word, made a correct response to an instruction, or turned toward the door when it has suddenly opened. However, unless the patient consistently responds correctly in this manner, that is, unless it can be proved that it was a response given other than coincidentally, the patient cannot be recorded as having achieved that level of ability. Relatives and others with a strong emotional attachment to the patient can all too easily believe that a coincidental sound or movement is a voluntary act.

It is important to remember that, because of spontaneous recovery, the level of stimulation given during nursing procedures, visitors' sessions, and the stimulation you have provided, an evaluation is almost invariably 'out-of-date' as soon as it has been completed. Why, then, evaluate? The results of an evaluation provide a base on which to plan treatment, and are useful in providing information on problems which may emerge.

The therapist must 'be continuously alert and sensitive to changes in his level of responsiveness and in his emotional and neurological state' (Carr and Shepherd, 1980).

Recording information is very personal, and what one therapist feels comfortable with another may not. Whether records are kept in note form, translated into graphs or flow-charts, or kept on assessment sheets, they must be clear, concise and in a language which is universal and meaningful. The author likes to record details which may appear to be of little value, but become very useful when reviewing the case at regular intervals.

FAMILY INVOLVEMENT

The family of a head-injured patient is as affected, more in some ways, as the victim; therefore they should be given due consideration. In the early days, very little of what you say may be remembered, much may be misunderstood, and statements may be remembered out of context.

Everyone must take care to repeat important information, to encourage relatives to ask questions, and in this to be consistent with all other team members, to take one day at a time, and to be supportive without raising unrealistic hopes and expectations. This is very difficult for all concerned.

If there is any information which the relatives particularly need to remember, the spoken word should be reinforced by the written. Careful consideration also needs to be given regarding information about local support groups (for example Headway in the UK). If presented too early the information may not be retained, and if too late a vital source of support will have been unavailable at a crucial time.

If we are aiming to work initially with the patient for several short sessions a day, one of these sessions should involve the relatives, the reasons for including them being:

1. To give them confidence in handling and touching the patient.
2. To encourage them to approach the patient in the correct manner.

3. To give a sense of purpose to the visit; so that they will feel not helpless but helping.
4. The patient will often respond more positively to a familiar voice.
5. To increase rapport between staff and patient's relatives.
6. To provide support.

Education of the relatives is important when one considers that it is they who are with the patient, not just during the day, but during the evenings and weekends, and it is through the relatives that a rehabilitation programme can be maintained, and approaches remain consistent. This is not to suggest that the systems generally adopted in hospitals – of rehabilitation staff working five days a week – is realistic in the treatment of head-injured patients, but it is the system which exists, and it will exist for the foreseeable future. It is the relatives who are going to be, in many instances, responsible for continued care and rehabilitation in the community. The relatives are key workers in the treatment of their head-injured relatives at all stages. Having said that, in hospitals where resources are stretched, it is not uncommon for relatives to take over the care of the patient to the extent that they are helping not only with rehabilitation, but also with nursing. Nevertheless, a distinction needs to be drawn between including them in the therapeutic team and abusing their readiness to help. All this is commendable, but, without guidance, education or support, efforts are inevitably misplaced and may handicap recovery.

ENVIRONMENT

The head-injured patient's environment is important to his rehabilitation programme, but it is often difficult to control.

Intensive care unit

Following injury, it is probable that the patient will be in an Intensive Care Unit (ICU) where rehabilitation staff will be doing the ground-work before treatment, and in some instances, starting treatment.

Research on the effects of an ICU's environment on the wide range of patients admitted has shown that it is often a source of psychological stress (Tomlin 1977; Chew, 1986). Tomlin found that over half of the patients who stayed in an ICU developed simple reactive depression, usually after five to six days and lasting for seven to 10 days, showing signs of apathy, lack of co-operation with staff, and fall in morale causing possible deterioration in his physical condition.

Whilst Tomlin and Chew were concerned with the numerous clinical conditions which necessitate this type of environment, we cannot dismiss the adverse effects when considering the head-injured patient. Although the patient may be unresponsive, or heavily sedated, there may be those who have fluctuations in levels of awareness, or who remain in ICU for long periods because of an unstable medical condition or the presence of serious associated injuries.

Tomlin also found that increased attendance by relatives did not reduce these effects – patients gained substantial emotional benefit from relatives' visits only whilst they were present.

In his study, Chew noted that over half the patients complained of sleep disturbances and of pain. Hallucinations appeared to affect some patients, but these were thought to be hypnagogic, that is, in the state between wakefulness and sleep. Tomlin noted that a much rarer, but much more serious, disturbance sometimes occurred when the patient was being weaned from the ventilator and had to sleep for the first time without support. Bentley *et al.* (1977) at St. Mary's Hospital found that the noise level in an ICU during the day was equivalent to heavy street noise. These findings do indeed suggest that ICUs are a source of psychological stress.

With the head-injured patient in coma or in stupor, we need to normalize sensory input and control stimulation sources. Because of the nature and intensity of care given in an ICU, a patient can easily be regarded as an object of treatment, rather than a human being. In addition, normal sensations are removed, for example a catheter takes away the normal sensation of urination, and a nasogastric tube removes the sensation of eating and drinking. The patient will be touched at regular intervals for the purpose of examining and recording and for basic needs. Some equipment makes slow, rhythmical, monotonous sounds, and the lights may be on for 24 hours so that the patient will have no indication of night and day. Thus 'an already damaged system is further deprived of necessary sensory input' (Farber, 1982).

Although there is increased awareness of these disturbances and efforts are being made in many units to keep the patients in touch with reality (Stratton, 1988), an ICU is not an ideal environment in which to commence a stimulation programme because of the inevitable distractions. However, because it should be assumed that the patient can hear until it is proved otherwise, general nursing and essential physiotherapy can be used for stimulation by accompanying these activities with clear words of explanation, orientation and encouragement.

Hospital ward

On progressing to a less intensive care ward, the principles are initially the same – returning the patient as far as possible to normal and avoiding excessive stimulation. This is very difficult in any sort of ward.

The surroundings need to be interesting enough to induce the patient to keep his/her eyes open; they should include isolated, familiar objects in strategic places. The space over the patient's head should not be forgotten; for those who cannot imagine how boring a hospital ceiling can be, try lying still and supine on a hospital bed for a while. A simple mobile is an acceptable accessory over the bed (as long as it is related to the patient's age) and it will be a valuable focusing aid.

Avoid cluttered bedside cabinets, walls and surroundings which 'flood the system'. If there are visual problems the patient will be better able to recognize his/her own possessions if they are isolated against a plain background.

Sounds should be controlled so as to allow the patient the opportunity to attend to those that are meaningful. There appears to be little point in playing music to the patient for long periods because it soon ceases to be a stimulation; stimulation will occur when it is turned off!

Treatment environment

The environment for evaluation and treatment at this stage should be quiet, so that stimulation can be channelled. It need not be a sound-proof room but one in which outside noise is reduced or absorbed by soft furnishing. Ideally, this area needs to be near to the ward so that the patient can be transferred with the minimum of fuss, and also so that help is near at hand if it should be needed.

Positioning of the patient within the environment

How the patient is to be nursed deserves consideration; for example should the patient be nursed on a bed, on the floor, in a hammock or deckchair, or a combination of these? No possibility should be ruled out and the ultimate decision needs to reflect the individual needs of the patient and requires regular review. Naturally, the hospital's system must be flexible enough to allow divergence from standard practices.

Nursing a patient on cushions on the floor in an enclosed area has the advantage of allowing the patient to move around should he become able to do this. Restraints are unnecessary because the patient cannot fall and injure himself. Staff must approach at the patient's own level, which helps to remove some of the barriers between staff and patients. Physical therapy is aided by the patient being in a position suitable for mat work.

However, being on the floor is not a customary position for an adult and may hinder the processes of visual perception as the patient will not be seeing objects, people or actions from a usual position. This nursing position also complicates moving the patient from lying to sitting, and increases handling of the patient for reasons of correct position prior to feeding, washing, toilet or therapeutic activities.

Some patients feel more comfortable and secure in a bed with retaining sides, and may be content to lie still whilst resting. Other patients may be frustrated by being enclosed and may have to be restrained from hurting themselves either by climbing over the bed sides, or by banging limbs against them. Physical restraint of patients needs to be avoided because it can increase frustration, aggression, and agitation.

It is easier for the patient to start to practise dressing whilst on the edge of the bed, and transferring from a bed to a chair is easier than transferring from the floor to a chair.

A hammock or deckchair can be of value in breaking down extensor spasm or posture. Tilt-back chairs, deflatable duvets and moulded seating may be advantageous for day use, depending on tolerance, level of awareness and treatment plan. Positioning of patients is further discussed in Chapter 5.

The entire treatment team should be in agreement as to the positions of nursing, treatment and leisure to be adopted. Health and Safety regulations still apply and must be complied with.

STIMULATION PROGRAMME

The stimulation programme is not something which is conducted primarily by one individual for set periods each day; it should be carried out by the entire treatment team, including relatives, during contact with the patient wherever that may be, and at times when he will be most responsive.

However, as with any person recovering from a severe illness or injury, it is necessary for there to be adequate periods of rest, which means that stimulation needs to be carefully controlled if it is to be of value.

Nursing should be seen a part of this programme, with careful words of explanation, orientation and encouragement accompanying any act however often it may be performed. It is important to name the part of the body that is being worked on, to describe what the patient should be feeling, and to encourage an appropriate response to that stimulation.

The approach to any head-injured patient should be appropriate to age and status and this should be understood by all, including relatives and visitors who come into contact with the patient. This particularly applies to ward cleaners, who take all sorts of patients to heart.

Although some members of the treatment team are concerned with the patient's physical requirements, others are concerned with the stimulation programme. The author aims to see the patient daily for three periods of between seven and 10 minutes each and to increase this as tolerance improves. Timing is important in that it should not follow any tiring activity in which the patient has been involved. These planned sessions are the ones the author shall be emphasizing, although, as mentioned above, the programme should involve all persons coming into contact with the patient.

During treatment sessions, if possible, the patient's trunk should be upright because this enables him to view the world around him from a normal position, provides a more familiar sensory input, and allows him greater opportunity to respond to the environment and the therapist.

Because we always assume that the patient can hear until proved otherwise, nothing should be done to the patient without slow, clear words of explanation, orientation and encouragement. It should become a habit every time one approaches the patient at the beginning of a session to introduce oneself, tell him where he is, what day and time it is, and to where you are taking him and what you are going to do.

The injured brain depends for its recovery on stimulation and activity, as does the immature brain for its development. Ayres (1979), found that if the visual system is damaged, visual stimulation is necessary and, likewise, if there is damage to the auditory centre, the brain needs to experience noise in order to organize auditory functions. Vestibular and tactile stimulation, however, is seen to have effects throughout the whole of the nervous system.

Deliberate and therapeutic stimulation is the beginning of the process of restoring the integrative action of the nervous system; this is because the patient's reaction to it creates his own source of stimulation. In practical terms, the patient should be encouraged to respond appropriately to the stimulation, and, indeed, to environmental influences.

The stimulation should, as far as possible, be familiar to the patient, hence the importance of knowing as much about the patient as possible. Different sorts of stimuli can be combined but be aware of 'flooding the system' by using too many at the same time (Bartholomeus, 1975). An example is washing: one can soap a body part, the patient can smell it, and the activity can be accompanied by a verbal explanation of what the patient is feeling and smelling.

All stimulation should be broken down into component parts, with well-timed input and ample time for the patient to respond.

Touch

Contrasting stimuli, such as hard and soft, hot and cold, rough and smooth, can be used on many parts of the body and should always be accompanied by clear words of explanation, orientation and encouragement. The stimuli used should be familiar and relevant to the individual patient.

The patient should be given ample time to respond, be encouraged to localize the stimuli, to move away from painful and otherwise unpleasant sensations and to react appropriately to pleasant ones.

As far as possible, avoid causing abnormal patterns of movement and increase in tone.

Temperature receptors are found all over the body but it would seem that there are more 'cold' areas than 'warm'. 'Warm' receptors discharge at a steady rate when the skin temperature is between 35°C and 45°C. Sudden heating of the skin will produce a rapid surge of impulses, but this tends to be short-lived. 'Cold' receptors discharge at a steady rate at a skin temperature between 10°C and

35°C. Sudden cooling of the skin will also produce a rapid surge of impulses.

If using ice for stimulation, do not leave it on the skin for too long because it can damage the skin and adaptation will occur – the stimulus no longer provides a discharge from the receptors and it will no longer act as a stimulus. Do not use ice near the mid-line of the body and be cautious when using it around the mouth as this may set off a seizure in those with a tendency to seizures (Zoltan and Meeder Rykman, 1985).

Continuing pressure on some parts of the body can have a calming effect. When upset, many people will press their lips in an effort to control emotions; others may hold something to them (such as a cushion), putting firm pressure on the abdomen; others may press their hands together. Firm, constant pressure on these areas, as well as to the soles of the feet, may have a general calming effect on the patient (Farber, 1982, pp. 126–8) and should be used when a patient's general agitation is distracting his attention from therapeutic processes. The therapist must be sensitive to the changing state of the patient so that she/he takes the patient only to a point where he is receptive to therapeutic stimulation, and not to a point from which it is going to be difficult to rouse him.

The guidelines for observation during evaluation should be followed for recording of responses in treatment.

Hearing

Patients should be given clear, simple words of explanation, orientation and encouragement, and we should initially be finding out if the patient can localize sound and follow simple instructions. Note that turning the head to locate sound is, initially, an automatic rather than a voluntary response.

Use sounds which are familiar to the patient, for example relatives' voices, dogs barking, clapping hands, jingling bells, telephones ringing, and favourite music. One of the most remarkable examples of the value of the familiar and purposeful that the author has seen was in a patient who had been totally unresponsive until the author accidentally put on the record-player, at the wrong speed, a 'single' that the patient had recorded as a professional entertainer. On hearing this at the wrong speed the patient quickly located the sound and became increasingly agitated until the speed was corrected.

23

The fact that sound can excite or soothe should be used to promote a desired state in the patient. Soft, melodic music is restful, but loud, powerful music is excitatory. Your own voice can be used either to elicit movement by using short sharp commands, or to relax the patient by talking in soft tones.

With this knowledge, auditory stimulation can be carefully controlled, generally beginning the session with excitatory sounds (unless the patient is very agitated), and ending with soothing ones so as not to leave the patient in an agitated, anxious, or restless condition.

Sight

Opening the eyes may be facilitated by stroking the lids in an upward direction and holding them open for a short period. This should be accompanied by clear words of encouragement. On the opening of the eyes, the patient must be presented with an object of interest in order to gain or maintain attention. This can be a familiar person, for example a relative; a familiar belonging; a mirror if there are no facial injuries or change of features (a shaved head); or a brightly coloured disc, which can be verbally associated with common objects, for example yellow can be associated with the sun, daffodils, or a bedroom at home.

Once the eye fixes on an object one should try to lead on to tracking an object from side to side and up and down. The objective is for the patient to attend to his/her environment and gain control over visual stimulation by self-initiating tracking of an interesting object/person, and by self-regulating the current object of interest.

Smell

Smells familiar to the patient may be used as stimuli, either in association with other senses or with no more than verbal associations.

The smell receptors adapt within seconds or minutes depending on the substance – this is known as 'olfactory adaptation' (Keele *et al.*, 1982). When this occurs, the intensity of the odour has to be increased in order to excite the adapted receptors. Whilst wishing to use strong odours, whether pleasant or unpleasant, the first exposure must be to a diluted form with subsequent exposures increasing in strength. McCormack (see Pedretti, 1985) recommends using solutions of 30% strength, followed by 60% and then full-strength, in order to extend the working time.

Adaptation is selective, and, although it has occurred with one odour, another will produce normal sensations. Nevertheless, a rest period of 30 seconds should be given between successive odours in order to prevent masking of new stimuli.

Substances which activate the trigeminal nerve as well as the olfactory should be avoided: these include ammonia, camphor, aniseed, menthol, cloves and peppermint (Gordon, 1982).

It is possible to purchase odour kits and coma kits, which include natural smells of sufficient strength to be of value in a sensory stimulation programme. However, the author prefers to use fresh items with naturally strong odours that can be incorporated into the individual treatment plan according to familiarity. For example odours of onion, coffee, washing-up liquid and furniture polish can be used with a patient whose prime occupation is housewife; leather can be used with a patient who enjoys horse-riding; brush and hand cleaners can be used with the patient who is a painter and decorator. Although collecting one's own odours for stimulation is preferable, it does require considerable imagination on the part of the therapist.

Taste

Do not begin stimulating taste buds until you have tested the swallowing and gag reflexes to see if the glossopharyngeal and vagus nerves are intact.

Sweet, salt, bitter and sour solutions, such as sucrose, sodium chloride, quinine, vinegar and lemon-juice, may be used, and patient's facial and postural changes noted. One can use fine tweezers to place minute amounts of a solid on the tongue, or, if the patient is able to swallow, an eye dropper, swab or small muslin-bag may be used to deposit a substance in the appropriate part of the mouth. Caution should be practised, however, particularly in the presence of a bite reflex, and in creating excessive salivation. The patient's reaction should be carefully watched.

SUMMARY

Early intervention has been shown to significantly reduce the total rehabilitation period, mainly by maximizing the potential for recovery, by avoiding medical complications, by controlling the environment, by preventing behavioural problems and by facilitating early education of the family in the process of rehabilitation.

Early intervention can be practised in any hospital, given some ingenuity in applying the principles to the individual patient and the available surroundings.

Evaluation is essential before commencing the stimulation programme, and this involves looking at the physical, sensorimotor, visual and communicational elements. The medical history has notable implications for rehabilitation and outcome and should be considered carefully in the process of evaluation.

The relatives should be seen as key workers in the programme of treatment and there is a need for early introduction to the rehabilitation process. Remember that the family is as much affected as the injured person, and therefore they require considerable support, guidance and encouragement from all the persons involved.

The environment often has at first to be organized to allow the patient to react to it without 'flooding' the system with excessive stimuli. The therapeutic use of the natural environment should be encouraged as soon as possible.

The programme of stimulation should not be regarded as treatment that is separate from the daily routine, but an integral part of it. All activities should be accompanied by clear, concise words of orientation, explanation and encouragement. One should assume that the patient can hear until proven otherwise.

A given stimulus can be used for different effects, depending on how, when and where it is applied. However it is used, the patient's response must be carefully noted. It must be remembered that differences in response occur according to such variables as mental development, sex, age, fear and anxiety, and previous experience.

Thought should be given to the sequence of stimulation: it may be necessary, initially, to use stimuli which will arouse the patient, but one does not want to leave the patient in an agitated state. Avoid using too many similar stimuli as this might cause a rebound affect. For example too many calming techniques may cause the body processes to speed up in an attempt to restore homeostasis.

Duration of perception does not necessarily match the duration of stimulation; perception of the stimulus may last beyond its application or it may rapidly decrease during application (adaptation). Adaptation varies with each sense. According to Gulbrandsen *et al.* (1972), when the same noise stimulus is presented daily to an unconscious patient, the patient adapts to the noise over a much shorter period on successive daily applications. They concluded that if there is a response there is habituation. However, a study by Bjornaes *et al.* (1977) on response habituation using touch, concluded that there was little evidence to suggest that habituation did, in fact, occur in the unconscious patient.

A programme of stimulation should not be started with those patients who have raised intracranial pressure, are on artificial ventilation or who are highly sedated. Additional injuries may also contra-indicate treatment initially, and it should be in consultation with medical staff that priorities in treatment should be determined. Additional injuries may also prevent one from carrying out methods of restoring normal sensory input and rule out some methods of stimulation. In such cases the therapist's priorities should be to prevent functional disability, to adapt the environment to suit the needs of the patient, and to educate the family in the process of rehabilitation.

The ultimate object of the sensory stimulation programme is to enable the patient to react as normally as possible to the natural environment, by encouraging self-regulation, as well as self-initiation of stimulation sources.

3

Activities of daily living

Activities of daily living are those, such as washing, dressing, feeding, which most of us carry out without help in order to maintain our personal level of care. To perform these activities without help is the difference, to a disabled person, between being independent or dependent (Turner, 1981).

The unconscious patient is dependent on all those around with responsibility for his/her well being, and, as his/her awareness improves, the very passive participation in a 'normal' daily routine will be a step towards independence.

Taking the patient through the movements of being dressed, fed and washed is part of the programme of stimulation, as well as having a valuable influence on physical and cognitive abilities, and on orientation to reality. If these activities are to be incorporated in a programme of treatment, they must be carried out at the most appropriate time in the day, every day, and they should be carried out by the same person – consistency is very important.

As the patient improves, more should be expected from him/her – a passive role should be gradually replaced by an active one in pursuit of independence. When a form of communication has been evolved, the patient should make such decisions as which shirt to put on or whether to have ice cream or custard for dessert.

With daily practice, those patients with potential will be able to relearn skills or adapt tasks in order to become independent. What we must be aware of is that, unlike victims of other injuries, the head-injured patient may have difficulties of a very diverse nature including initiation of movement, disorders of motor planning and perceptual problems. Some patients are labelled as lazy when in fact they cannot, rather than will not, co-operate in treatment. Before reaching this conclusion, the patient should be properly assessed in the specific areas related to performance.

The dictionary's definition of 'rehabilitation' is 'to restore to former position or rank' (*New Collins Concise Dictionary*, 1985). There are many other definitions of the word in the medical sense but it must be recognized that recovery from severe injury of the brain is often incomplete and in some cases lifelong care, of one kind or another, is necessary. The word 'rehabilitation' is too much used to be discarded and may properly be regarded as a process that may never achieve its end but should not be abandoned.

As members of the treatment team we must be careful not to impose our own standards on the patient thereby making our aims and objectives unrealistic in the light of the patient's needs and desires; we must look positively at what she/he can achieve and not devalue this by comparing it to the performance of an uninjured person.

With the severely head-injured patient, using everyday activities as a therapeutic medium is very time-consuming because it is necessary to give words of explanation, encouragement, and orientation, as well as physical promptings, opportunities for rehearsal, and ample time for the patient to respond. Apart from these difficulties, in a general hospital there may be other barriers to the effective setting of a daily routine. Among these are interference with or by the hospital's own daily routine, team members' responsibilities to other patients, staff shift systems (and Monday to Friday working week for rehabilitation staff), incontinence, lack of adequate clothing, physical, perceptual, and behavioural disorders. However, through allowing flexibility of the 'system', training and guidance for the relatives, and shared responsibility and communication between members of the treatment team, the difficulties can be overcome.

REALITY ORIENTATION

In Chapter 2 we discussed the need to alter the environment in order to restore normal sensory stimulation and to help to orientate a confused patient. The environment must give the patient clues to the time, place and person; and, by setting up a daily routine as close to that followed at home, we are treading a familiar path towards reorientation.

As well as being given clues to orientation, the patient must be enabled to respond appropriately. For example activities such as washing, dressing, and feeding performed in the ward by others encourage the patient to do the same. The environment can also be organized to orientate the patient by providing a clock, calendar, and familiar items of interest and relevance, whilst observing all the precautions relating to flooding the system with too much information.

Introducing oneself as one approaches the patient, providing orientation information at the beginning of each task (making links with environmental clues), should be followed throughout the period of disorientation, both day and night, and by all members of the treatment team, including relatives.

As the patient regains awareness of his surroundings, she/he is likely to be disorientated. Because of this lack of understanding of where and perhaps who she/he is, the patient may display bizarre, meaningless and aggressive behaviour which may be hazardous to him/herself or those attending him/her. Alternatively, the response may be that of apathy. Whatever the reaction, the disorientation needs to be reduced by careful adaptation of the environment and acknowledgement of the patient's difficulties.

If disorientation persists, consideration needs to be given to labelling the resources of daily living such as 'bed', 'lounge' or 'bathroom', with words or symbols. Colour-coding routes to bathroom, treatment and leisure areas may be necessary, and the keeping of a timetable and diary by the patient may help in the process or reorientation. Where the patient can read and understand it is necessary to ensure that newspapers/magazines left for him/her are up to date and that the calendar is changed daily.

The therapist needs to keep pace with the constantly changing needs and abilities of the patient and to adapt the amount of prompting given to help orientation. The patient must learn to use his/her initiative and reasoning ability in picking up clues to orientation.

THERAPEUTIC APPLICATION OF EVERYDAY ACTIVITIES

The head-injured patient's dependence on others for personal care is not related only to the level of consciousness, but also to the limitations in physical and cognitive abilities. Because patients have such diverse needs, the combinations of which are often unique, it is impossible to give other than general guidance in this section.

Factors which determine how activities are to be carried out include age, sex and culture, as well as previous personal preferences. The level at which the activity is currently performed depends on the conscious level, degree of physical and cognitive impairment, the patient's behaviour, tolerance to activity and the degree of active involvement by the family or other members of the team. The balance of activities performed during the day should be determined by his tolerance of demands made on the patient's time and energy.

The primary evaluation of the patient's ability will be the base-line from which to work, and the component parts of each task need to be identified in order to assist the patient. As the patient begins to respond more appropriately to the sensory stimulation programme, or to simple commands, she/he can be encouraged to carry out simple, automatic, self-care activities. These activities can be initiated by simply giving the patient a tool and an instruction, such as a tissue and a request to wipe his/her mouth after dribbling. Many actions may be automatic to the patient, although she/he may not be able to initiate these tasks without prompting. It is all too easy to let the patient assume the sick role by doing everything for him/her, when in fact, with correct prompting she/he is able to carry out more than is expected.

The tasks to be carried out by the patient need to be structured at a level which allows the patient to succeed in them. This requires careful attention by the therapist to the patient's constantly changing state and needs.

During the performance of tasks, the patient's responses need to be carefully noted in order to identify difficulties which may not be easily noticed in the performance of one task, but appear consistently in one or more others. Early acknowledgement of these disorders may enable the therapist to adapt the activity to help the patient to overcome the difficulty. Helping the patient to overcome his difficulty, by whichever way the activity is approached, may reduce the patient's frustration.

The Rivermead ADL Self Care Scale (Whiting and Lincoln, 1980) was devised to assess recovery in patients with hemiplegia following cerebral vascular accident. Research has shown that return to independence is on a progressive scale, and, as the brain recovers in much the same way whether injured by vascular accident or a blow to the head, further studies indicate that the scale can be applied to the head-injured population.

The expected order of recovering the ability to look after oneself is as follows:

1. Drinking.
2. Cleaning teeth.
3. Combing hair.
4. Washing face and hands.
5. Making up or shaving.
6. Eating.
7. Undressing.
8. Indoor mobility.
9. Moving from bed to chair.
10. Going to the lavatory.
11. Outdoor mobility.
12. Dressing.
13. Washing in the bath.
14. Getting in and out of the bath.
15. Overall washing.
16. Moving from floor to chair.

Although return is expected to be in the above order, it does not mean that the patient's personal priorities should match. Order of activities should be determined by the current aims of treatment, reality orientation programme and daily routine adopted.

It is up to the members of the treatment team to decide, according to the experience and judgement of the individual therapists and the needs of the patient, what the plan of treatment is to be. The team needs to be divergent in reasoning, display great imagination, perseverance and initiative as they draw from all areas of knowledge according to the problems with which they are faced. However, the individual approach to the patient needs to be consistent in order not to confuse him.

I realize that it should go without saying, but the patient's dignity should be preserved wherever possible, and whatever the level of consciousness, the patient should be treated with respect, and privacy should be maintained in the performance of the more intimate parts of personal care.

WASHING

Initially this is used as part of the stimulation programme. As the patient begins to respond more appropriately to his/her environment and to commands, she/he should be expected to become more active, starting with automatic actions such as wiping the face with a face-cloth after initiation by the therapist, to initiating and executing this activity without prompt.

Practical considerations

Environmental considerations

The degree of dependence will depend on the level of consciousness, as well as other disabilities. Washing can initially take place sitting in, on or by the bed, progressing to the bathroom if there is sufficient privacy for the patient as well as others wishing to use it. This activity should be carried out at the most appropriate time of the day with due regard to the previous personal habits of the individual patient.

In order to elicit the best performance from the patient, she/he should be comfortable in the environment. Washing may take considerably longer than when carried out by an uninjured person, so the area must be warm; it must be remembered that discomfort caused by being cold or having a full bladder, or incorrect seating, etc., can increase any spasticity, and impair concentration and co-operation. If the patient feels hurried by the therapist, this will also affect performance. A noisy environment may also be distracting to the patient and so should be controlled as far as is possible.

Physical considerations

To mitigate physical disorders, a good sitting position should be achieved, according to patients' needs and set objectives, as well as appropriate placing of the bowl, and towel and so on. The amount of support given in sitting will be determined by the patient's need for it.

The therapist should be in a position to give the support and encouragement needed, giving the patient sufficient security to perform difficult tasks. Movements which will lead to increase in tone in affected muscles, or reinforce incorrect patterns of movement should not be encouraged. Techniques taught should be in accordance with the patient's individual treatment plan. Observation of the patient in, and discussion with the staff of, physiotherapy or occupational therapy departments will give guidelines for positioning the patient in sitting (whether this be on the edge of the bed in a static seat or in a wheelchair) and in transferring from one position to another. Work with the patient under supervision initially if you do not feel confident in the physical aspects of this work, as lack of confidence will communicate itself to the patient.

Purposeful activity achieved by the patient should always be appropriately rewarded; this can be with word, gesture or token – whichever is meaningful to the patient.

Disability equipment

While the patient is disorientated or confused, it is not advisable to introduce disability equipment, such as a wash-mitt or suction nail-brush, as these may only confuse the patient more. The use of a mirror, as well as verbal and physical prompting, may be all that is required to elicit automatic movements.

As the patient becomes more orientated in time, place and person, the introduction of necessary disability equipment may be made in order to gain independence in this activity.

Perceptual considerations

Visual perceptual deficits can be mitigated by keeping the work area uncluttered, making sure the face-cloth is of a different colour from the wash-bowl, and the towel a different colour from the surface it is to be found on. Verbal accompaniment can reinforce other visual components, such as spatial relationships, body image and left/right discrimination, i.e. 'the soap is *under* the face-cloth' or 'dry your *left* hand'.

If there is neglect of one half of the body, stimulation of the affected side can be conducted in an attempt to make the patient aware of it. This may be attempted by the therapist sitting on the affected side so as to encourage the patient to acknowledge it (training in scanning across the mid line). While encouraging the patient to watch, wash the neglected side, giving clear words of explanation and orientation. Encourage the patient to do the same thing with his/her unaffected hand whilst watching. A mirror may help when performing this activity, although it is not always recommended. This is a 'sensory integrated approach' much favoured in the treatment of children with defective perception. However, more research needs to be carried out on its effectiveness in adults.

A more favoured approach by therapists to the treatment of perceptual disorders is that of practising tasks, and this is seen by the patient as practical and understandable. This is commonly known as the 'functional approach', which allows for compensation for a disability and treats the symptom instead of the cause. Although the patient may learn to wash him/herself through practice aided by verbal and physical prompting, the perceptual disorders she/he may experience will still be apparent in other activities, unless they are also practised in order to compensate (Sieve and Freistat, 1976).

There are many other aspects of perception to be taken into account, too many to be covered in this chapter, and it is recommended that you refer to Chapter 4 for further information. Staff and relatives should be kept up to date with the patient's level of independence so that they can keep pace with the patient's recovery and provide continuity of care.

DRESSING

Although significantly low on the scale of expected return to independence (Whiting and Lincoln, 1980), dressing is an important part of a daily routine and serves as a boost to morale, if not for the patient, then for the relatives.

Physical barriers to independence in dressing are easier to overcome than cognitive barriers – one can teach new methods, provide disability equipment and adapt clothing. However, there may be many reasons why the patient is unable to carry out some stages of dressing and these reasons may be very complex.

Generally, it is easier for the patient to participate initially in undressing, and backward chaining may be very helpful for retraining: that is, for the patient to always be active in the last part of undressing yet to do a little more in each session until independent. By this method she/he always has a sense of achieving something. The same method can be adopted for dressing.

The patient needs to be reminded throughout the day about his/her state of dress so that she/he becomes increasingly attentive to his/her appearance. One should aim at the standards adopted before the accident and recognize that interest in dress will improve as the patient becomes more perceptive and thoughtful with an increasing appreciation of dignity.

Difficulties may arise because a patient is not fully continent. Although it is much easier to deal with a patient who has a catheter in place, this is increasingly unacceptable as orientation improves and there is increasing need for the patient to learn to control his/her sphincters. In striking a balance one should perhaps err on the side of optimism and accept the risk of an occasional accident with the need to have spare clothing available.

Practical considerations

Environmental considerations

The environment should be warm, comfortable and private and one in which the patient feels secure. Dressing should follow on from the washing activity and should therefore be conducted in the same place with the same amount of support from the environment and from others.

Reality orientation

Dressing is an important part of reality orientation due to the visual nature of the clue for differentiating between night and day; people dress in the day time and wear pyjamas or nightdresses at night. It is important that this activity is done at the most appropriate time of the day.

Cognitive considerations

Poor attention span, distractability, disorientation, poor understanding of language, and poor short-term memory cause many difficulties for the therapist and patient. Much prompting, both physical and verbal, will initially be needed to redirect attention. Particularly with the agitated or restless patient, the therapist should make the most of periods of more or less calm and understanding.

Dressing practice must stimulate the patient to reason out the process of dressing rather than allow him/her to rely on the directions of the therapist; most of us have seen a patient who, when left to his or her own devices has, for example, put both lower limbs into one leg of his/her underpants and has not been able to work out how to correct this, if, indeed, he/she has recognized it as needing correction.

Even if the patient is unable to carry out any part of the process of dressing, she/he should be encouraged to make decisions about what clothes to wear, for example the red shirt or the blue shirt. It may be very difficult for the patient to respond to such a request and it may take all her/his efforts to indicate a preference. How she/he relays the decision will depend on the system of communication which has been adopted.

Physical considerations

The natural sequence of dressing after washing may result in an unacceptably long period of treatment and the therapist must not overtax the patient's tolerance.

For the confused patient, the use of disability equipment will only serve to confuse him/her further, and poor short-term memory will be a barrier to learning new techniques. At this stage the patient will need continual prompting to redirect attention to the task in hand, and to discourage incorrect or unwanted patterns of movement. Diversionary tactics may need to be employed if the patient begins to show frustration, and consequently withdraws co-operation. The therapist needs to adopt a carefully balanced approach to the needs and mood of the moment, but not lose sight of the eventual goal.

If not able to stand, the patient should feel confident in the seating arrangements, which should allow adequate movement and access to clothes. Confidence is perhaps the best foundation for a determined effort. The therapist should be in front of, or to the side of, the patient depending on the degree of assistance needed, or behind him/her if he/she is continually asking for unnecessary help.

Encourage the patient to start from the top and work down, as far as possible to do everything sitting, and to keep shoes on (except when putting clothes over feet) to aid standing when this is necessary. A mirror may be a help in dressing, but attention may need to be directed to unfastened buttons and neglected parts etc.

Choice of clothing

Clothes should be easy to get on. Track suits, if normally worn by the patient, are particularly useful as there are no fastenings, they are loose and comfortable and allow ease of movement. Under-garments, shirts, trousers, jumpers etc., should be chosen for comfort, as well as uncomplicated fastenings. Any fastenings should be large and accessible to the patient, at the front instead of at the back. Females should be advised to wear trousers rather than skirts or dresses, in the interest of modesty during the demanding daily programme.

The most suitable garments are easy to clean, hard-wearing, and crease- and stain-resistant. Relatives should be encouraged to accept responsibility for regular cleaning of garments. Alternatively, a member of staff may do this. The hospital laundry can be used if personal clothes are not likely to get lost and if the patient has the necessary reserves of clothing. When able to do so the patient may wash his/her own clothes, if necessary, under the supervision of a volunteer.

Disability equipment

As the patient becomes more aware, equipment such as long-handled shoe-horns, elastic shoe-laces, dressing-sticks and so on, can be introduced. It may be beneficial to adapt the clothing by incorporating Velcro fastenings or front openings or to add loops to zips. New techniques can be taught and encouraged as appropriate. In the interests of consistency in methods of good dressing, all team members should be kept up to date, and the order and methods of dressing should be listed and kept in the dressing area. Even with a consistent approach, the patient may insist on adopting his own method according to previous habits or because of ease of results. Those methods adopted may not be the methods prescribed by the therapist but may have to be accepted if one is unable to gain the patient's co-operation in practising new techniques.

Loss of use of one side of the body

Techniques for retraining hemiplegic patients to dress are well documented (Eggars, 1983; Trombly and Scott, 1977; Pedretti, 1985; Turner, 1981), but procedures adopted will depend on associated disability.

Even before retraining begins, the patient should be given responsibility for her/his own extremities and encouraged to move the affected limb(s) with the sound arm. For example, with the aid of the sound arm she/he can place his/her affected limb in the sleeve of the shirt during assisted dressing.

Incorrect patterns of movement should be avoided or carefully controlled to prevent them from becoming habits. There is a danger that patients will feel that any active movement of the affected side is better than no movement, no matter from where that movement is initiated. As well as avoiding incorrect patterns of movement, the emphasis should be on avoiding associated reactions, maintaining muscle length, maintaining symmetry of the body and improving the function of the affected side (Eggars, 1983). All treatments should be planned to bring the affected side into action, whether for holding or supporting or for more complicated functions.

Perceptual considerations

Independence in dressing is dependent on such perceptual abilities as intact form constancy, figure/ground, spatial awareness, as well as absence of apraxias or agnosias. Careful records of the patient's performance during dressing should be kept and analysed in relation to the results of tests of perception.

The presence of sensory impairment and communication disturbances (both expressive and receptive) should be considered, as these may affect the patient's performance and may be misinterpreted as perceptual dysfunction.

The following are points to consider in facilitating independence:

1. Keep the area uncluttered.
2. Avoid placing clothes on the same coloured surface, for example do not put a white shirt on a white sheet.
3. Choose clothes that are plain – patterns distort outlines.
4. Choose clothes that have large, simple and few fastenings.
5. Think about how to present the clothes, preferably they should not be in a muddled mass.
6. Clues may need to be added to the garments to indicate the back/front, left/right, inside/outside. Labels, coloured thread or other marks may be used but should not be obvious once the garment is on.
7. Use a mirror to prompt dressing of a neglected side.
8. Patients may find it useful to use a list of the order of dressing; symbols or words can be used.
9. Give verbal reinforcement throughout, depending on nature of perceptual impairment; 'your shoes are *under* the chair', 'put your *left* arm in the sleeve' and so on.
10. Be consistent in the timing, sequence and general method of dressing.

CONTINENCE

Control of the bladder and bowel is a complex act which is disturbed following severe head injury. Incontinence and retention result from disturbance of the afferent or efferent pathways between the brain and the viscera, or of pathways within the brain itself. In some cases of retention, dribbling (retention with overflow) of urine may be misinterpreted as incontinence.

Coma removes voluntary control of the bowel and bladder which is not necessarily restored as consciousness returns. Some patients need a great deal of help in regaining control of these organs.

Initially, it is nurses who assume responsibility for the care of bladder and bowel as part of the general care of the patient and it is probable that within the hospital or within the health authority, a nurse will be designated as adviser on incontinence and give advice on suitable appliances and other methods of treatment.

Therapists contribute to the management of incontinence by adhering to the system adopted by the nursing staff, and by not interfering with the function of appliances as by kinking tubes or accidentally removing them. Much can be done to disguise appliances in order to maintain the dignity of the patient, for example by attaching catheter bags to the inside of clothes rather than leaving them showing.

Dispensing with appliances should be regarded as part of the programme of treatment and training that is worked out by the team and maintained throughout the 24 hours.

Points for consideration when incontinence occurs

1. Incontinence may not result from damage to the brain but from associated disorders or complications, such as infection.
2. The type of incontinence: dribbling, stress or urgency (Mandelstam, 1977), and times of incontinence (particularly of faeces) should be noted. If a regular pattern is seen, consider implementing a training programme, for example hourly, two-hourly, or before or after events such as meal times, bearing in mind the fact that habits of urination or defaecation vary greatly from one individual to another.
3. The patient may try to escape from unwelcome experiences by being regularly incontinent, for example at the beginning of a treatment session, or when a task becomes too difficult. Always be prepared for such an occurrence and deal with it with as little disruption to the treatment session as possible.
4. The patient may be incontinent because of the pleasure derived from having genitalia exposed and touched. If so, be as impersonal as possible during the cleaning-up procedure, and, wherever possible, this should be performed by someone of the same sex as the patient.
5. If the patient has been incontinent during a session, think back to see if there was any indication that the patient wanted to pass

urine or faeces. Did the patient show signs of discomfort or was she/he more than usually distractable? Did the patient try to communicate his/her immediate needs to you? If so, inform other members of the treatment team how she/he did it.

6. A disorientated patient who can get out of bed may be unable to find a bottle, commode or lavatory. This type of patient may urinate or attempt to do so on or near other patients' beds, in corners or in wardrobes, etc. The environment in this case should be provided with reminders, labels and/or signs that the patient can easily recognize and the nearer to the lavatory the better.

7. Is the patient periodically incontinent because she/he is unable to attract anybody's attention to help him/her to a commode or lavatory? If so, can the patient find out or be shown how to attract the attention of an assistant when the need arises, and if so without the embarrassment of making his/her needs clear to all and sundry.

8. Is the patient periodically incontinent because it takes too long to undo clothing? If so, more suitable clothing should be worn. For example, tight trousers with difficult zips and buttons can be replaced by loosely fitting 'jogging' trousers. French knickers have wide legs, which can be pulled aside for urination, and can replace tight fitting knickers. Open-crutch knickers can also be considered.

9. Make allowances for disorders of perception, for example if the patient neglects one half of the visual field, make sure that the urine-collection bottle is within the used field of vision; even then, however, the patient may fail to recognize it.

10. Incontinence of either urine or faeces is very embarrassing for the patient who is aware of the significance. Never take the patient from the ward without a change of clothing if he is in the early stages of retraining bowels and bladder. Any accidents during treatment sessions should be dealt with as quickly as possible and with little fuss. This helps morale, as well as wasting as little time as possible.

11. If a patient has worn an appliance for some time, dispensing with it may cause anxiety; for example, the patient may want to make abnormally frequent visits to the lavatory, and if prevented from doing so may become increasingly agitated and distracted. This problem needs to be dealt with according to the individual needs, but, generally, little attention should be drawn to it and one may hope that the adjustment period will be short and that

the patient will gain confidence in his ability to hold his water. If incontinence persists, the reason needs to be identified and suitable steps taken to remove it.

12. Patients may need training in getting on and off the lavatory seat or commode, and training in cleaning themselves after urination and defaecation. The team will need to be consistent in the method adopted so as not to confuse the patient, and will need to be in harmony with the physical and cognitive abilities, as well as with the hospital and home facilities.

13. The disability equipment which may be needed can be a raised seat, frame, urinal (female or male), and appliances to hold toilet paper during use (if the patient's level of awareness is adequate). When the patient starts going home, any appliances used should be available there.

FEEDING

Nutritional requirements of an injured person are considerable and an adequate, as well as a balanced, diet is necessary. A severely head-injured patient can lose between 10 and 40% of body weight, with recovery of this loss taking up to a year (Berrol, 1983).

If the patient is unable to swallow either liquids or solids, she/he will require tube feeding, but this is unpleasant and may cause local irritation; it also prevents the normal sensations experienced during eating and drinking. It is important, therefore, to retrain swallowing as early as possible in order to effect the removal of the nasogastric tube.

If any reflexes are found to be abnormal, or there is any doubt as to the ability of the patient to cope with consuming liquids or solids, a speech therapist should be consulted. She/he is in a position to assess the situation, and recommend further objective assessment, for instance video fluoroscopy, or recommend a pre-feeding programme which should be closely followed.

Because training and experience are required in facilitating inhibition techniques, these are not included in the text, but the author strongly recommends the practice of caution. Dieticians should also be involved, whether the patient is independent in feeding and/or drinking or not, in order to ensure she/he receives an adequate diet.

Even with patients who do not have difficulties in eating and drinking, caution must initially be practised and the following points taken into consideration.

Positioning

As far as possible, the patient should be upright with the head in the mid line. Initially, the feeding programme should be conducted in a quiet environment where the patient is able to attend to the therapist without distraction.

Consistency of food

Semi-solids are easier to swallow than liquids. When possible, therefore, liquids should be thickened by freezing and 'slushing' and some foods, for example bananas, can be puréed. The therapist must be sensitive to the changing abilities of the patient; a prolonged semi-solid diet will not encourage biting and chewing (Warner, 1983).

Whole milk products thicken oral secretions and so should be avoided early on in the feeding programme. Sweet solutions will increase saliva production and should, therefore, be avoided in dribblers.

Acceptability of food

Do not force patients to accept food they do not normally like or eat. (Refer to individual personal history sheets.) Home-cooked food that has been puréed is preferable to most hospital soft diets, and will cater for the individual preferences.

Facilitate swallowing and chewing

Gentle rotary movements, by finger(s) under the chin, with firm pressure upwards will elicit tongue movements and thereby encourage swallowing. Follow this by gentle stroking along the chin and down the throat. Avoid the Adam's apple, as this may cause choking.

To encourage chewing try circular motions, using the fingers and thumb, around the cheeks.

Precaution

Ensure that the mouth is empty after feeding; otherwise the patient may later choke. As a further precaution, and with regurgitation in mind, it is wise to keep the patient upright for at least 30 minutes after feeding.

Tidy habits

When the patient is able to swallow liquids, encourage the use of a cup instead of a feeder as this is more normal. Aim for a high standard by drawing the patient's attention to dribbling and spilt food and encourage him to dab, rather than wipe, this away himself.

Relearning movement patterns

The difficulties of feeding may not be anything to do with chewing and swallowing, but arise from difficulty in getting the food to the mouth because of physical or cognitive defects. To relearn the physical aspects of feeding, the patient may need to be taken through the relevant actions accompanying this with clear words of explanation and orientation. Backward chaining may be appropriate in many instances; encouraging the patient to complete the last part of feeding first, for example:

1. Take the spoon out of the mouth.
2. Push the spoon in the mouth, take the spoon out.
3. Lift the spoon to the mouth, push in and take out.
4. Scoop food, lift spoon, push in mouth, take out.

Disability equipment

Cutlery can be adapted to meet the needs of the individual patient; handles can be enlarged and straps may be used to secure utensils. The patient should become independent with a spoon before she/he progresses to a fork and then to a knife. Non-slip mats prevent a plate from moving around the table, and plate guards prevent food from being pushed over the edge (such an obvious aid as a plate guard should, however, be dispensed with as early as possible). If the patient is very slow in feeding, provide a heated dish in order to prevent food from getting cold and unappetizing.

Perceptual considerations

To reduce the effect of any visual perceptual problems which may be present, keep the table clear of any clutter, provide only the utensils for immediate use, and provide food which is clearly identifiable on a plate and which does not run or blend into neighbouring foods. Although the patient should be given a selection to choose from, the foods should have distinctive flavours and textures in order to aid identification and tempt the patient (within the given guidelines).

SUMMARY

Activities of daily living are those everyday tasks necessary for looking after ourselves. By incorporating everyday activities into treatment, we are initially enhancing the stimulation programme, as well as having a useful influence on the patient's physical, and cognitive recovery.

Only the basic activities of washing, toilet, dressing and feeding have been discussed; the principles underlying them can be applied to other activities of daily living relevant to the individual patient.

The establishment of a daily routine is necessary to the process of reality orientation, and familiarity helps to give the patient the confidence she/he requires. If everyday activities are to be used, they should be carried out at the most appropriate time of day, in the most appropriate setting. One must work to the patient's previous standards and not impose one's own, but one may have to be content with what can be done rather than deploring how much less than normal it is.

The team needs to be consistent in its approach to the patient, to be divergent in its thinking, and must display great imagination, perseverance and initiative. The team has to be sensitive to the constantly changing needs of the patient and should be careful to communicate this.

The therapist should be aware of his/her own limitations and request help from colleagues as appropriate: one may initially need to work on patient transfers, i.e. chair to bed, under the supervision of a physiotherapist, and those without training in the process of feeding should follow the direction of the speech therapist. One cannot be expected to be knowledgeable and/or experienced in all methods of care.

Everyday activities are understandable to relatives and they may feel able to participate in promoting independence. They should be educated in the methods used and encouraged to take over certain tasks, particularly in the evenings and at weekends. Some relatives will be unable to watch the patient struggle to dress or feed himself, and, if this persists, they should be temporarily diverted to help in tasks with which they are able to cope.

4

Perception

The *New Collins Concise Dictionary* (1985) defines perception as 'the process by which an organism detects and interprets information from the external world'.

Merely to experience sensations is not sufficient to interact effectively with the environment: the sensations must be organized, interpreted and stored so that, ultimately, we build up a complete picture. We rely on interpretation of stimuli to satisfy our needs, to warn us of impending danger, to anticipate events, to interact with objects and people, to give us pleasure and so on. By means of stored information, gained through past experience, man becomes very efficient at recognizing objects, people and places with the minimum of sensory information (Foss, 1966).

Perceptual difficulties may result from head injury and are generally associated with damage to the non-dominant parietal lobe. The more common head injury is diffuse and produces less clearly defined disorders of perception than can be expected after localized injury. Any disturbance of one or more perceptual ability may result in disruption of function, confusion, agitation, bizarre and meaningless behaviour, or apathy. Defective perception may be confused with motor problems, lack of co-operation, poor motivation, or behavioural disturbances; it should be acknowledged as soon as possible so that the therapists' approach can be determined, and the environment and resources adapted to allow compensation.

Assessment of perception may be difficult due to decreased awareness, poor concentration, distractability, expressive or receptive language difficulties, or physical disability. Subjective, as well as objective, assessment is valuable, particularly in the early stages, and previous intellectual level, cultural background, sex and age, should all be taken into consideration.

ASSESSMENT

Objective assessment of the perceptual state of the patient should be conducted by a psychologist, and in his or her absence, by an occupational therapist. However, it is necessary for all team members to have a basic understanding of perception, and of the effects of perceptual dysfunction.

The experiences and observations of all team members are valuable in determining the nature of deficit(s), if this has occurred following injury. The patient will react differently in different situations, at different times of the day, and during interaction with different people. Unless the members of the team discuss their separate findings, their partial understanding of the patient's difficulties may lead to incomplete and perhaps conflicting attempts to overcome them. For example: four weeks after severe head injury, a child was examined by members of two disciplines and diagnosed as having severe hearing impairment. However, earlier in the day the child had been painting in the occupational therapy department and had carefully followed the verbal directions of the therapist who had stood behind her. This demonstrates the need to assess carefully the whole picture, co-operate on a team basis, and systematically analyse each presenting symptom.

When working with, or caring for, the patient we must ask ourselves:

1. What can the patient do?
2. What can the patient not do?
3. Does she/he carry out activities on instruction, to imitation, or without prompting?
4. What prevents the patient from achieving success in a familiar task?
5. How does the patient respond to failure to complete a familiar task?
6. Does the patient's performance improve under different conditions?
7. Is the patient consistent in what she/he *fails* to do?
8. Does the patient fail to attend to things on one side of the body, or fail to attend to things generally?
9. How does the patient move around?
10. How does the patient respond to excessive noise, hands on, or 'busy' visual stimulation?

In a busy ward, it is easy to overlook vital clues because a number of the people involved with the patient's basic care are also responsible for the care of others. It may also be that relatives, or untrained personnel in the course of their duties, inadvertently conceal evidence of defective perception, for example, by clearing away plates with half the food left on them or helping in personal care by ensuring that the last slipper is on the foot, or the arm put in the sleeve. Such help is given with the best of intentions and the need for it is not reported.

When one has asked the pertinent questions regarding the patient's performance, one may find that some pattern has emerged that occurs in all activities attempted, or that difficulties arise only under certain conditions. One needs to remember that an observed abnormality may have more than one cause.

More formal tests of perception are available of both standardized and non-standardized sorts but, interestingly, a study by Ottenbacher (1980) of the work of occupational therapists in this connection, indicated that the majority tested by clinical observation. When studying the schools of thought on perceptual dysfunction, one can see that the more formal approaches may over-simplify the problem, and concentrate on quantity rather than quality (Abreu and Toglia, 1987); they may determine the presence and severity of the disorder but reveal little about the patient's everyday performance (Lezak, 1983). A patient may not perform as well in tests as in natural activities – as many examination candidates are well aware.

According to Abreu and Toglia (1987), it is not sufficient to have 'yes' and 'no' answers for tests of function; it is necessary to know how the patient went about accomplishing the tasks. The methods can in turn be analysed. This approach takes into account the cognitive components of function, and selective, as well as generalized, treatment can be adopted at the relevant level.

Formal assessment is necessary in order to evaluate systematically and objectively the patient's abilities and disabilities, establish priorities in treatment, monitor improvement, and evaluate methods of treatment. A common language is needed in order to communicate the patient's disabilities to other members of the team. Measurements are a necessary, if not always reliable, basis for comparison. Further work is needed to formulate both cost- and time-effective functional assessments.

In order to carry out the more formal assessments, such as the Rivermead Perceptual Assessment Battery (RPAB), or the Chessington O.T. Neurological Assessment Battery (COTNAB) (both of which are for adults), the patient should be sufficiently alert and orientated to be capable of attending to such tasks. Ideally, assessment batteries should be completed within one session, or at most, within two.

Other evaluation manuals guide the therapist through mainly unstandardized tests of perceptual dysfunction in adults (for example Sylvester, 1973; Sieve and Freishtat, 1976; Ontario Society of Occupational Therapists' Study Group, 1977).

Most of the standardized tests of perception have been developed for use with children. Such material requires considerable modification if it is to be applied to adults who have generally acquired a fund of knowledge which is stored in long-term memory. The material designed for young developing minds (emphasizing the development of new skills) may not be easily applied to the brain which has already developed those skills (Abreu and Toglia, 1987).

Preliminary steps

1. Determine the patient's level of orientation, memory, attention span, reasoning, and insight.
2. Determine the patient's previous level of intellectual ability. The use of the Mill Hill Vocabulary Scale Synonyms Test, National Adult Reading Test, or the Graded Naming Test is recommended in the Rivermead Perceptual Assessment Battery; alternatively relatives may be able to provide this information.
3. Determine if the patient wore glasses or a hearing-aid. If used, these should be worn by the patient during assessment.
4. Determine the existence of any visual defects, such as hemianopia or double vision.

   Homonymous hemianopia

   This is loss of vision one side of the mid line and is caused by blindness in the lateral (or temporal) half of the visual field in one eye and loss of the medial (or nasal) half in the other. In effect, a patient with left homonymous hemianopia will not be able to see anything to his left unless he turns his head, and vice versa (see Figure 4.1). Many patients will compensate for this loss automatically, whilst others will have to be taught to do so. The visual fields are tested by having the patient seated before one and fixing his/her gaze on the end of the tester's nose. A finger is then moved towards the mid line first from one side and then the other and the patient is asked to say when

Figure 4.1 The visual field loss in homonymous hemianopia. Many patients automatically compensate for this loss of vision and others can be taught to do so: (a) left homonymous hemianopia; (b) right homonymous hemianopia; (c) smaller lesion may give rise only to a quarter of the visual field as in this upper homonymous quadrant.

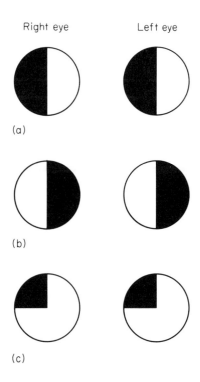

Right eye   Left eye

(a)

(b)

(c)

it comes into view (see also the section on visual extinction).

Diplopia
Double vision is a fairly common complaint in the early stages after head injury and the patient may gain some benefit from wearing an eye patch but it should not be worn continuously or always on the same eye. If double vision does not recover spontaneously, the patient learns to compensate.

5. Determine abilities in receptive and expressive language, as some tests depend on the use of language. Refer to the speech therapy services for assessment.

6. The patient needs to feel confident and comfortable in an upright

position. Voluntary control of one or both hands is generally required for completing tests of perception.

7. Assessment, at every level, should always take place in a controlled environment.

VISUO-PERCEPTUAL DISORDERS

It has been estimated that normally approximately 90% of information about the world around us comes through our eyes (Foss, 1966). Visual field defects are common after severe head injury and whilst many of them will recover spontaneously, some may last for a long time. The visuo-perceptual state requires regular reviewing and the programme of treatment should be regulated according to current difficulties and the patient's ability to co-operate.

Initially, the patient is observed for his/her ability to track an object across the mid line and up and down, and the quality of movements is noted, as well as what attracts the patient (see also the section on initial evaluation guidelines in Chapter 2).

As the patient begins to respond more effectively to stimulation and to instructions, she/he can be given tasks which indicate her/his ability to recognize colour, shape and size. These activities may include: pointing to different stated colours or shapes; pointing to the biggest or smallest; classifying shapes; drawing shapes; matching colours or shapes (form constancy); pointing to, or picking up, familiar objects; matching objects with pictures. These tests should require only simple, basic responses from the patient and they can be carried out with the minimum of equipment at little or no expense. With imagination, these can be altered to exclude the use of language.

The therapist should be aware of the possible existence of specific visuo-perceptual problems and assess accordingly as the patient improves.

Visual extinction

Visual extinction is the failure to acknowledge a stimulus when a similar one is presented at the same time in the corresponding half of the visual field; the stimulus is recognized if presented on its own, in any part of the visual field (Walsh, 1978). Extinction can occur in any of the sensory modalities.

Visual agnosia

Visual agnosia is the failure to recognize a familiar object through sight, when the problem is not caused by sensory impairment or intellectual deterioration. In cases of visual agnosia, the object may be recognized through the other senses, for example by touch.

There are several subdivisions of visual agnosia; **visual object agnosia** is failure to recognize an object for what it is, or failure to recognize a pictorial representation while still being able to describe it accurately. An interesting example of this has been given by Sacks (1985), when after examining a glove a patient described it as, 'A continuous surface infolded on itself. It appears to have five outpouchings, if this is the word'. There was no recognition of it as a glove until a clue was given and he accidentally slipped it onto his hand.

A patient with visual object agnosia may be able to use the object even though she/he fails to recognize it, but would be unable to describe the function of an object when shown it. This differs from nominal aphasia in which the function of an object can be described but not named. The patient can be assessed by asking him/her to point to named objects and to demonstrate their use. Realistically, this assessment should make use of normal activities, such as feeding or dressing.

Prosopagnosia is the inability to recognize faces, even of relatives and in some instances, even one's own, although the individual features are recognized and it is known that it is a face. In some reports, it is suggested that people experiencing this difficulty may recognize faces by prominent characteristic features (Sacks, 1985). It is rare for poor recognition of faces not to be accompanied by visual field defects.

The patient can be tested by being shown photographs of familiar people and asked who they are, and also by watching his/her response when a relative approaches, to see if there is recognition without verbal prompting. The patient can be given visual clues to recognizing individual members of staff. When in the bathroom, or during washing and dressing activities, check if the patient can identify him/herself in the mirror.

Figure/ground discrimination

Figure/ground discrimination is the ability to distinguish by sight an object or figure from a competing background. Common examples of this disorder are the inability to find a glass on a crowded locker, a pen in a cluttered drawer, or a white towel on a white sheet.

How the patient manages in his/her surroundings will give some indication of difficulties of this sort. The patient can be asked to select a named item from a group of three or four on a table, but the therapist should be sure the patient knows what to look for. Ask the patient to identify the individual foods on the plate at meal times (although this is not always easy with hospital food!). Observe him/her during normal activities, such as identifying clothes to put on, or locating soap to wash with.

More formal assessments involve asking the patient to draw around embedded geometric shapes and to identify embedded objects in a complex picture. An example of this type of assessment is the Southern California Figure-Ground Visual Perception Test (FGP), which is designed for children. Peterson (1985) found that this was also reliable when used on adults; the scores tended to be stable between the age of 15 and 45 years but performance declined after this. Although there is some disagreement about it, it appears that males perform better than females in figure-ground tasks when they require a motor response.

VISUO-SPATIAL DISORDERS

Visuo-spatial disorders refer not to problems of the recognition of objects but of recognizing their position in space, and their relationship to oneself or to other objects. This may include difficulties in dealing with concepts, such as up and down, in and out, behind and in front, and in discriminating between left and right, and in estimating distance, depth, or direction.

We require visuo-spatial skills in order to deal effectively with the environment, particularly in movement. Without the ability to estimate location of objects and relationships between objects and self, and without the ability to perceive distance, depth and direction, we are a danger to ourselves, for example when crossing a road, or with open fires and electrical appliances.

Difficulty in judging depth and distance may alarm the patient; for example, when standing she/he may feel much further off the ground that she/he is and be reluctant to stand or move about for fear of falling.

Position in space

Awareness of position in space deals with the concepts of in and out, up and down, behind and in front and can be tested by watching the patient follow instructions such as finding his/her shoes *under* a chair, or putting the spoon *inside* the cup. In the kitchen, one can ask the patient to put the milk-bottle *behind* the sugar, or the mug *next* to the plate.

The author uses a set of photographs containing a spoon inside, behind, in front, to the left of, and to the right of a cup; and a woman behind, on, in front, to the left, and to the right of a chair. The patient is asked to point to the picture indicating a named position. The actual objects can also be used, for example ask the patient to put a spoon in certain positions relative to a cup.

Spatial relationships

Spatial relationships are concerned with perceiving the position of two or more objects in relation to *oneself* and in relation to each other (Sieve and Freishtat, 1976).

The patient should be observed in normal activities. If she/he can get about observe how she/he moves, particularly around obstacles, and note how she/he goes about standing, walking, climbing stairs. Observe the patient when sitting from standing; can she/he judge distance? When a bean-bag or ball is thrown at the patient; does she/he grasp too soon, or does it hit the patient before she/he moves to catch it?

When she/he is washing or dressing, hold necessary articles in front of the patient so that she/he has to reach to take them. At meal times observe the patient picking up the fork, putting salt on the meal, or pouring water into the glass. Does she/he over reach, under reach, or overfill the glass?

Construct simple two- or three-dimensional patterns and direct the patient to copy these. They could include a series of patterns made up, initially, of two components and increasing in complexity as the patient accomplishes more. The patient should be given five or six components from which to select. They could be wooden-blocks or pieces of cardboard. The patient's ability to manipulate the pieces into the correct position should be noted, for example is she/he able to turn a triangle around in space to match the example pattern?

Use lollypop sticks to make simple designs for the patient to copy (these are easier to handle than matchsticks). Mark two series of six or eight dots on a table between the patient and the therapist, one series for the therapist to work on and one for the patient. Ask the patient to watch while you connect a selection of dots in a simple pattern, then ask him/her to copy. Take note of the patient's strategy for completing this task (see also the section on the Frostig Developmental Test of Visual Perception).

Unilateral visual neglect

Unilateral visual neglect involves the ignoring of visual events on one side of the body's mid line (usually the left). This can occur with or without hemianopia and it may be accompanied by unilateral tactile and auditory neglect (see also the section on hemi-inattention).

Topographical disorientation

Topographical disorientation means that the patient has difficulty in understanding the relationship between one place and another. If mobile, she/he may have difficulty finding her/his way from the ward to the occupational therapy or physiotherapy department, or from a side room to the bathroom, even though she/he may have followed this route many times. This problem exists in the absence of memory problems or confusion.

During daily movements, do not lead the patient from one place to another, but request him/her to direct you. At corners wait for him/he to tell you which way to turn and if the patient can get about, keep behind him/her so that he/she receives no clues about the route but can receive help and guidance if a wrong turning is taken. Topographical disorientation may also be a problem in familiar areas in and around the patient's home.

TACTILE PERCEPTION

The first things to record concerning reactions to touch are whether responses are delayed, absent, localized or generalized. The duration of the stimulation should also be noted. As the patient becomes more responsive assess the following: light touch, firm pressure, and superficial pain. These can be tested by stroking small areas of the hand with cotton-wool buds; pressing firmly with a finger tip on the same areas of the hand; and pricking these areas with a pin. The patient should not be able to see what is happening. Hiding the parts being tested behind a screen is preferable to blindfolding. If the patient feels the contact she/he should be asked to point to the area stimulated and also asked if it feels the same as a corresponding normal area. The results should be recorded on a visual chart.

Heat and cold can be tested with four test-tubes filled with water at obviously different temperatures. The patient should be able to say how they compare with each other.

Proprioception

Proprioception, or positive sense, enables one to recognize, by feel, the movement and position of parts of the body. Testing involves covering the eyes, gently supporting a limb, and gently moving a joint by 5° to 10°. The patient is asked to indicate if she/he feels a movement, and, if so, in which direction, and in what joint. Do not place your fingers in the plane of movement: they should be across it so that there is no clue from the pressure exerted by them. Do not use abrupt movements, or those which stretch the muscles, tendons, and joint capsules because pain can influence proprioception (Eggars, 1983).

Asterognosis

This is the ability to identify objects by touch, in the absence of sensory loss. With vision occluded, the patient is asked to identify, by feel, such common objects as a spoon, safety pin, or penny. Each hand should be tested separately and the different test objects should not be handled in the same order.

If the patient is unable to name the objects, ask him/her to describe them. Prevent auditory clues by padding the area on which you are working – dropping an object on a hard surface may identify that object.

OLFACTORY AND GUSTATORY PERCEPTION

It is important to be able to identify tastes and odours, particularly if one lives alone or is responsible for the care of others. If one cannot do so, one is in danger of not detecting gas leaks or burning, one cannot know that food has gone off and one cannot identify substances in unmarked containers etc.

Without adequate taste and smell, the reduced enjoyment of food may lead to eating too little.

Olfactory perception

This can be tested by using substances such as coffee, almond oil, peppermint and musk. Do not use ammonia, acetone and menthol because they stimulate the trigeminal nerve, and can be perceived even by those with a total inability to smell (Gordon, 1982).

Different substances should be presented to the patient in identical containers. Ideally, three strengths of the substance should be available (see the section on olfactory stimulation in Chapter 2), so that if the patient does not initially recognize the smell a stronger solution can be presented. If the patient cannot explain what he can smell his expressions and other reactions may indicate that he is at least aware of a smell.

Gustatory perception

The ability to perceive taste should not be tested unless the swallowing and gag reflexes are present (see the section on gustatory stimulation in Chapter 2). Use only sweet (sucrose), salt (sodium chloride), bitter (quinine), or sour (lemon), for testing taste because many substances can be identified by smell (Westerman et al., 1981). Use a cotton-wool bud to place the substance, mixed with a drop of water, on the tongue. It should be identified within 5 seconds.

According to Weiffenbach (1982), the ability to taste salt and bitter declines with age, but this is not the case with sweet and sour.

BODY SCHEME

Body scheme is knowledge of one's body parts based on sensory information from within and outside the body. It encompasses perception of body position and the relationship of body parts, and is the basis of motion – we need to know our body before we can hope to gain control over it. **Body image** is different from body scheme in that it expresses one's feelings about one's body and does not represent the physical structures.

Somatognosia

This is a disturbance of body scheme involving the lack of awareness of body parts, failure of recognition of parts, and failure to recognize their relationship to one another. The ability to dress oneself is poor if disorders of body scheme exist; one cannot expect a patient to put clothes onto a limb if he is not aware of the part, or does not recognize that part in relation to the rest of his body. Other activities of daily living may also be impaired.

Warren (1981) looked at disorders of body scheme and constructional apraxia in relation to predicting failure to become independent in dressing following cerebral vascular accident. The results indicated that, although there was significant correlation between tests of body scheme and constructional apraxia, body scheme was a more reliable predictor of independence in dressing.

Simple tests for body scheme, other than observation, include:

1. Asking the patient to point to parts of the body.
2. Asking the patient to imitate movements performed by the therapist.
3. Asking the patient to draw a person, assemble a felt figure, or assemble a face from given pieces.

Anosognosia

This is a lack of awareness of the existence of disease or disability sufficient to cause it to be denied or misinterpreted, as in the case of a patient of whom it was reported that 'When he woke up he felt fine until he moved in the bed. Then he found, as he put it, "someone's leg in the bed – a severed human leg, a horrible thing!" . . . at this point he had a brainwave. He now realized what had happened: it was all a joke – a rather monstrous and improper, but a very original joke!' (Sacks, 1985). Anosognosia may accompany hemiplegia, hemianopia and hemianaesthesia (in conjunction or separately).

This condition may be detected in the course of conversation, or everyday activities. Conversation may reveal unrealistic attitudes or confabulation and these are more likely to be detected if the patient is encouraged to speak about his or her disability.

Anosognosia can influence motivation during the rehabilitation phase – the patient will see little point in therapy if she/he does not believe that she/he has a disability.

Confusing left and right

Knowledge of left and right can be demonstrated by asking the patient to point to named parts of one or the other side of the body, or to pick up the spoon on the left, or put the shoe on the right foot.

Unilateral neglect

There may be a tendency to ignore one half of the sensory field of touch, sight and hearing. This occurs in the absence of sensory loss or weakness.

Typical examples of unilateral neglect are shaving only half the face, putting only one arm in a cardigan, and leaving the food on one half of the plate. When walking, the patient may constantly bump into things on the neglected side; in effect, she/he forgets that she/he has one side, unlike the patient with hemianopia who is more likely to compensate automatically for this disorder.

The concept of neglect is not only externalized. In some cases, if you ask the patient to imagine walking down a familiar street and ask her/him to describe what she/he sees, she/he may only describe the right side of the street. If this is the case, to get the same patient to describe the left side, ask her/him to imagine turning around and walking back down the street; she/he will then be able to describe the right side of the street which would have been the original unseen left.

Common tests for unilateral neglect include:

1. Asking the patient to draw a person and/or a clock-face. Parts may be missing or distorted on the left. Look at the quality of the work with regard to size, positioning, how parts are connected, and any undue emphasis (see Figure 4.2).
2. Asking the patient to copy a drawing of a house and/or a flower. The copy may be incomplete or distorted on the left (see Figure 4.3).
3. Asking the patient to mark the middle of a line. He may mark it a quarter of the way along.
4. If the patient can read, asking him to read a passage from a book may show that he fails to read words at the beginning of each line.

Figure 4.2 Asking the patient to draw a clock-face is a common test for unilateral neglect. Drawings may be distorted or have parts missing.

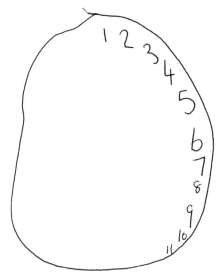

Figure 4.3 Asking the patient to copy a simple drawing of a flower may result in a distorted and/or incomplete picture if unilateral neglect is present.

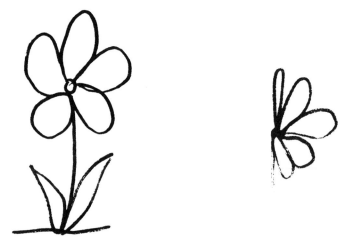

Drawing to be copied   Patient's drawing

Figure 4.4 Example of a felt figure of a man assembled by a patient with unilateral neglect.

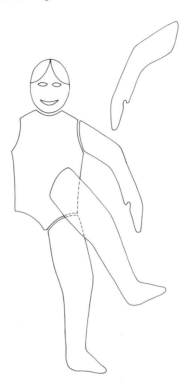

5. Asking the patient to assemble a felt- or card-puzzle of a person. He may fail to put on the left arm and leg, or put them in the wrong places (see Figure 4.4).

APRAXIA

Apraxia is the inability to carry out familiar and appropriate actions that is not the result of weakness but due to an apparent loss of memory of how to make certain muscular movements.

Different types of apraxia have been identified: constructional, ideomotor, ideational, verbal and dressing. Apraxia may occur with agnosia, dysphasia and disorders of memory and may occur singly or in combination.

Constructional apraxia

This is where the patient is unable to put together parts of an object to make a whole. It has a disordered organizational element which becomes evident in spatial aspects of construction.

Tests for constructional apraxia consist of drawing, copying and constructing, they include free-hand drawing, copying two- and three-dimensional designs. The interpretation of tests is complex, and dependent on the site of injury, and should, therefore, be objectively assessed by the use of tests such as the Rivermead Perceptual Assessment Battery, or Benton Three-Dimensional Constructional Praxis Test.

Baum and Hall (1981) looked at constructional apraxia as an indicator of dressing ability in the head-injured adult. They concluded that there was a significant correlation between dressing and constructional praxis, and suggested that testing for this disorder improves understanding of the patient's difficulties. It may be that if severe constructional apraxia indicates the inability to dress independently, or to *learn* to dress independently, the therapist will be able to concentrate her efforts on other priority areas of treatment.

Motor apraxia

Apraxia of this type may affect one upper limb, particularly the finer movements. If there is weakness in the limb, the clumsiness appears to be disproportionately great because of the loss of kinaesthetic memory patterns necessary for the formation of skilled movements.

Ideomotor apraxia

Difficulty in performing movements to instruction, even though the patient understands the task, is known as 'ideomotor apraxia'. Nevertheless, the movements may be carried out automatically. The patient who is seen to do tasks automatically when previously unable to complete them when asked, may be labelled as unco-operative by those who do not know of the condition. There may also be difficulty in copying movements.

Ideational apraxia

The inability to plan action and results in the patient's being able to carry out only parts of an action or to perform an action *similar* to that requested. Unlike a patient with ideomotor apraxia, one with ideational apraxia cannot describe an act but he can copy movements.

TREATMENT NOTES

Once the nature and degree of the patient's disorders have been established the team as a whole should decide the priorities of treatment. There are many variables which affect the approach adopted and these include age, sex, culture, previous intellectual ability, severity and combination of perceptual dysfunction, cognitive and physical state, degree of family involvement and home circumstances. Most importantly, the resources of time, personnel and expertise will have a significant impact on the treatment adopted. The question will inevitably be, how do we achieve the maximum within these considerable constraints?

When working with the head-injured patient in the early stages, we expect some perceptual disorders to recover spontaneously. Therefore, if we are aware of the difficulties she/he is experiencing, we can adapt the environment in order to help the patient to make some sense of his or her immediate world.

The fact that in the early days after serious head injury some degree of natural recovery from disorders of perception is to be expected, means that as far as possible the patient's position in the environment should be chosen so as to promote such recovery. As an example, if a patient who is completely unaware of the left side is placed in a ward with her/his left side towards the centre of activity, she/he is, to some extent, isolated because her/his source of stimulation is confined to the (right) wall and anything passing on the right or in front of the patient. However, adopting this strategy should not deter the therapist from efforts to make him/her aware of the neglected side. She/he should continue to sit on their left during treatment and always introduce necessary items, for example food, from this side and encourage relatives to do the same.

For those disorders which do not abate by spontaneous recovery, there is very little evidence to suggest that practice in a perceptual task will do any good. Because a patient improves on a set paper task this does not mean that she/he will automatically improve in a related functional task. It would therefore be negligent to concentrate on isolated perceptual disorders without tackling the more obvious and serious difficulties in accomplishing independence in activities of daily living. Paper or constructional tasks would also seem meaningless to the patient and may not gain his or her attention.

The policy many of us adopt is to practise a function, such as dressing, in the hope that the patient will eventually become independent in that task. But, again, we can ask ourselves if this is dealing with the actual problem. Abreu and Toglia (1987), believe that we should be looking into the cognitive strategies adopted in performing tasks and identify if the patient is actually attending to relevant features, grouping similar items together, formulating a plan, or breaking the task down into steps; this is why it is so important to watch what the patient does during activity. If we are able to identify an area of difficulty, it is possible that the patient can be taught a strategy to overcome this. This theory, however, is dependent on the patient being able to benefit from instructions and cues – the capacity to learn is normally reduced in the brain-damaged adult.

The patient, during normal activity, requires constant feedback as to what she/he is doing correctly and what, specifically, she/he is doing incorrectly.

One has to make use of what abilities the patient retains as a starting point for enhancing and extending them. Even if the patient does not understand, relatives and friends will recognize the value of using methods related to everyday needs.

Treatment considerations

The following notes are for the therapist to consider when faced with a patient with a perceptual disorder.

1. Adapt the environment in order to aid the patient in making sense of his/her immediate world. For example:
   a. In case of hemi-inattention, place the patient with his affected side to the outside of a group or room, so that she/he is not isolated in that situation.
   b. If the patient has hemi-inattention, make sure that the items she/he requires for independence, for example the urine-collection bottle, are within view.
   c. If the patient has difficulty in distinguishing an object from its background, organize the living or working area so that it is free from clutter. This applies particularly to the locker, drawer, and table. The patient will have a greater chance of

identifying important items in a well organized area.

2. Work in an undistracting environment for training purposes, so that the patient will be better able to attend to the task in hand, and the cues given to him/her.

3. Talk through what is to be done before the patient attempts to do it.

4. In everyday activities, supervise the patient so that appropriate cues and detailed feedback can be given. Be consistent in your feedback, but do not allow the patient to become frustrated and therefore unco-operative.

5. Teach the patient methods of checking to see if she/he has completed each part of the task that she/he was given.

6. The slow patient should be allowed to set the pace when carrying out a task. This is time-consuming for the therapist, but the patient should not be rushed nor should the task be done for him/her in order to move on to the next one.

7. One should try to make the patient aware of neglected parts of the body.

   a. Sensory integration techniques are popular, although there is no evidence to suggest that they are of value. An example of this technique is the rubbing of a neglected part, such as an arm, with a material, and explaining what the patient should be feeling. Ask the patient to watch while you do this and then ask him/her to do the same to himself/herself. Washing offers a good way of doing this because the sensations of wet and dry, hot and cold, rough and smooth can be exploited.

   b. Ensure that the neglected part of the body is within the patient's visual field. Always encourage the patient to move the neglected part with the sound limb. Make him/her aware of the precautions that must be taken regarding the neglected part, for example to make sure he/she puts a neglected foot onto the footplate of a wheelchair, and to make sure that it stays there, particularly when the chair is in motion.

   c. Practise putting body puzzles together, naming and pointing to the parts, naming and pointing to the left and the right ones. Use the therapist's body, as well as the patient's. With children practise dressing skills with dummies and dolls.

8. Visual, auditory and tactile extinction may be improved by practice in discriminating between the introduction of single and simultaneous stimuli.

9. With problems of visual neglect:

   a. Present all activities from the neglected side. Sit all visitors,

Figure 4.5 A letter cancellation task, which can be used to treat problems of visual neglect. Patients are asked to cross out all the letter As they can find.

```
G  D  D  F  A  H  T  C  A  J  U  L  A  B  A  C  D  Z  X  N
A  T  O  H  B  A  F  J  T  A  B  M  K  Y  A  X  H  L  T  A
D  F  G  A  R  B  H  O  A  F  C  V  D  A  X  M  H  V  T  V
B  A  L  A  R  H  F  C  A  C  A  H  Y  P  N  C  Z  F  N  A
S  B  J  A  B  V  G  T  A  M  K  I  N  A  K  L  J  H  G  F
A  C  B  G  U  J  M  K  A  X  H  N  A  V  B  H  G  T  A  U
```

especially those of considerable interest, on this side also. This will encourage head turning.

b. Work on scanning tasks, emphasizing the importance of head turning to the affected side, in order to look for 'lost' items. Use objects, blocks or letter cancellation tasks (see Figure 4.5), and make use of visual targets for the patient to work from, that is the patient must look to the affected side until he/she can see his/her target. The patient must be given adequate feedback during this activity.

c. In books, draw a bold, bright line down the left of each page and teach the patient to keep looking left until she/he reaches this marker before beginning to read the next line. Aim to train the patient to put his/her own marker, such as a finger or a clip, onto the page.

10. If the patient has a problem in visually identifying shapes, colours, size, or objects:

a. During normal activity, ask the patient to point to named colours, shapes, objects. Ask him/her to point to the *biggest* object, or to the *smallest*.

b. Ask the patient to feel, draw around, and colour in shapes.

c. Ask the patient to sort out blocks according to shape, size or colour.

d. To aid recognition of objects, ask the patient to feel the object while you talk about it, then look at the object while you talk about it. Quiz the patient by asking him/her to identify objects by sight.

11. If the ability to identify objects by touch is poor:

a. Use stereognosis games such as putting an object in a 'feely' bag (a cloth bag), and ask the patient to put his/her affected hand(s) in to identify it.

 b. Ask the patient to feel objects whilst looking at them, to associate what she/he feels with what she/he sees. Cover the patient's eyes and ask him/her to identify the objects.

 c. Rub different textures onto the patient's affected hand whilst describing what the patient should be feeling. Do the same to the unaffected hand so that the patient can make a comparison. Set tasks where the patient has to 'pair' textures without using his eyes.

 d. Teach the patient awareness of this dysfunction so that she/he can adopt ways of compensating for it.

SUMMARY

Perception is the process of organizing, interpreting, storing and responding to information received from one, or more, sensory organs: perception is required in order to make sense of, and interact with, our world. Disorders of perception can occur following head injury and may impair function, or cause confusion, agitation, bizarre and meaningless behaviour or apathy. Diffuse injury of the brain produces less clearly defined effects on perception than more localized injuries.

Early assessment is important because, although many disorders will show spontaneous improvement, we need to adopt the environment, and our approach, in order to aid the patient to make more sense of his/her immediate world.

The assessment should be carried out by all members of the team because the patient will perform differently at different times of the day, with different people and in different locations. Specific assessment should be conducted by the psychologist and the occupational therapist, either separately or together. The speech therapist must test for disorders of auditory perception because of its interrelation to language.

Subjective assessment is important, but one should be aware that any dysfunction demonstrated may be due to causes other than perceptual.

Strategies employed by the patient should be examined, and, if the patient is able to benefit from them, they should be encouraged. Strategies which will apply to all activities should also be encouraged. Specific cueing and feedback is required if the patient is to benefit from such a treatment approach.

The approach adopted will depend on the resources of time,

personnel and expertise. We must concentrate what is available on making the patient more independent rather than on actions with no particular part to play in everyday life.

5

Aspects of physical dysfunction

The physical dysfunction following head injury can be extremely complex and can tax the most experienced therapist. Because of the generally diffuse nature of the injury, the dysfunction may affect one or more limbs, increase or decrease muscle tone, be manifest in rigid states, limit the range of motion, produce altered reflexes, and affect co-ordination, balance, hearing, sight, and speech.

The possible combinations, and degrees of physical involvement, are endless, and may be in addition to general medical conditions (which may have affected the individual either before or after injury). Additional injuries may have been acquired at the same time as the head injury, and these may involve the chest, abdomen, spine and limbs.

Each head-injured patient is unique so this chapter can only provide broad guidelines for treatment. The reader is reminded that we each have our own area of expertise, and should be prepared to be guided through those areas in which we have little, or no, knowledge or experience. The physiotherapist should always be consulted regarding positioning and handling, and should work closely with the nursing staff who will, initially, be the professional group most concerned with the personal care of the patient.

Incorrect handling or positioning of the head-injured patient in the acute phase can result in increasing spasticity, contractures of soft tissue, decubitus ulcers, and respiratory problems. We need to remember that it is much harder to correct a deformity than it is to prevent one.

POSITIONING

Positioning in bed

Difficulties arise initially in positioning the patient because of possible related injuries, the presence of abnormal posturing or tone, the use of support and monitoring systems, and the patient's level of awareness.

If increased tone exists, the position in bed should inhibit this and prevent abnormal posturing, for example no muscle should be placed in a position of full stretch. The use of pillows, carefully placed to support limbs or prevent unwanted movement, can also prevent skin breakdown by reducing the risk of rubbing bony prominences.

If the patient is lying on his side, or is semi-prone, the shoulder girdle should be protracted and the elbows extended and supported on a pillow. The legs should be slightly flexed and parted by a pillow to prevent adduction and internal rotation. The feet should be supported in order to prevent inversion.

If nursed in the supine position, care should be taken not to increase extensor tone; this is avoided by placing pillows to break up the pattern, for example behind the knee, or to hold the head and neck in slight flexion. With retraction of the scapula, pillows will need to be placed under the upper arm to help to position the scapula in protraction. Foot-boards to maintain dorsiflexion are not recommended – the constant stimulation to the ball of the foot may cause an increase in any spasticity. The weight of the bedclothes should be removed from the patient, particularly from the lower extremities by the appropriate use of a cradle.

Positioning must be supported by careful and delicate handling of the patient during turning or other care processes, as pain or discomfort will increase any spasticity present. The physiotherapist will give advice on correct positioning for each individual, according to his/her needs, and also on turning and moving the patient – turning can be easy if done correctly.

It may be advisable to chart turning procedures and to provide a diagram of the positions to be adopted; these should be placed near to the bed so that all staff are aware of the needs of the patient and the techniques to be used.

Sitting

Because of the need to normalize sensory input, facilitate interaction with the environment, and inhibit abnormal muscle tone, it is important to move the patient from lying in bed to sitting in a chair early in his/her treatment. It will, however, be very difficult for the acute head-injured patient to maintain, or even achieve, good posture in sitting without considerable support.

The physiotherapist should initially direct this activity, ensuring that the handling of the patient is consistent with his/her needs. The occupational therapist will be able, with the physiotherapist, to assess the seating requirements and adapt the equipment to provide appropriate support for the patient, depending on the facilities and expertise available.

When the patient is initially moved from lying to sitting, pulse and respiration should be carefully observed for any indication of distress. The patient will be easily fatigued, and short but regular sessions of sitting will be preferable to longer ones. Care should be taken to co-ordinate sitting out with other activities, so that it is seen as purposeful.

Adapted seating

It is recognized that existing seating in general hospitals does not always lend itself to adaptation for the special needs of the head-injured patient (or that of many other cases). It is also recognized that the individual patient's shape, size and symptoms, are many and varied, so it would be impossible to stock seats for every eventuality. The head-injured patient may require adapted seating only in the early stages for a matter of days or weeks, and so it is impractical and unrealistic to order personalized seating from the relevant agencies until the long-term needs of the patient have been identified.

Therefore the most suitable seating available must be adapted. It is an advantage to have at hand a small supply of suitable seating which can be adapted quickly and easily, with a little thought and imagination. The following features are those which are considered to be of value and relate to both static chairs and wheelchairs.

Extended back (or head rest) in order to provide sufficient support for the patient, particularly of the head and neck.

The chair should allow tilting of the patient, initially to provide additional support for the head and neck. The tilt should not take place at the hips, for example the back should remain at right angles to the seat, and should not be at the expense of losing the chosen position of the patient. Ensure that tilting the chair does not render it liable to tip over.

The seat should be firm in order to provide a good base for positioning. Soft seats can be adapted using a board and firm cushion. Pressure relief cushions should be considered in order to avoid skin breakdown over bony prominences.

The chosen chair should have sufficient width of seating to allow for the patient's comfort, as well as ease of repositioning or moving the patient in and out of the seat. However, the seat's width should not be so large, in relation to the patient, that adequate support is not easy to achieve.

The seat's depth should be adjustable to allow those people with short thighs to attain 90° of knee flexion whilst keeping the hips at 90°. This can be achieved by fashioning inserts between the back of the chair and patient.

Lumbar, waist and chest supports may be necessary to achieve, or maintain, body alignment, and to prevent the patient from falling forward. A lumbar cushion may be necessary in order to support the curvature, maintain extension of the spine and promote better trunk control. If the chair does not have these attachments, its construction should be such that it allows for easy adaptation.

A pommel may be required to maintain abduction of the hip and to prevent the patient from slipping forward out of the chair.

Deflatable duvets are valuable in that, with correct use, they can help in adapting the most basic chair, and can take the place of lumbar and waist supports and of the pommel. Depending on the size of the patient and duvet, the support can also be extended to head and neck. The use of a deflatable duvet is limited as it can be used for short periods only; the patient will require repositioning every morning because the duvet will become soft after a few hours of use. Precautions need to be taken – if the duvet becomes soft when it is being used for support the patient will end up in a poor position, or may slide onto the floor. Duvets will become soft whenever air is introduced, for example as a result of punctures or inadvertent removal of the stopper. (It has been known for children on the wards to be inquisitive about the role of the stopper, and to experiment to determine the effects of its removal!)

Table attachments are useful in supporting the patient's arms whilst bringing them within his/her field of vision, and placing them in a suitable position to facilitate voluntary movement. At the correct height, the table will also provide trunk support, and, in doing so, encourage head control. The table also provides a suitable working surface for treatment activities.

Wide chair arms allow appropriate placement of the patient's arms in a spasticity-inhibiting position, in the absence of a table. These will also allow placement of a flaccid arm in a position of support, therefore relieving pain in the shoulder and arm, and preventing subluxation of the shoulder joint. As with the table support, correct placement of the arms will bring them into the patient's field of vision. Chair arms can be widened by fabricating attachable troughs or by purchasing an appropriate trough and cushion (Steed, 1986).

Foot-plates are necessary in order to correctly position the feet, knees and hips, provide support, and inhibit abnormal muscle tone. The foot-plates should be adjustable, and allow independent elevation of each leg. Removable foot-plates are a bonus because they help in moving the patient between a bed and chair.

It is definitely a bonus to have the chair on lockable wheels to assist in transporting the patient.

Attachments are required for necessities such as drip stand and catheter bag.

The chair needs to be sturdy, and designed in such a way that it is difficult, if not impossible, for the restless or agitated patient to tip it over.

The chair should have a stain-resistant surface, so that it is easy to clean. However, care should be taken regarding the surface on which the patient will be sitting, and this will differ according to whether the patient is sitting for long or short periods.

The greatest problem with adapted seating is that the more accessories supplied, the greater the chance of the parts getting lost, or not being used as intended. The moral here is to keep the adaptations as simple as possible and within everyone's capability. Labelling the removable pieces of the chair is always advisable.

Positioning in sitting

The pelvis

The position of the pelvis is the basis for good sitting posture as it will influence head and trunk alignment and alter tone in the extremities. Thus the pelvis should always be considered first.

The weight needs to be distributed equally through both buttocks and these should be as far back on the seat as possible. Help may be needed in attaining good flexion at the hips and a wedge cushion can be placed under the patient (the narrow end towards the back of the chair) in order to achieve this. The buttocks should be central on the seat.

In order to maintain this position, a hip strap firmly placed at an angle of 45° will prevent the patient from slipping forward, and will be quite comfortable.

Lower limbs

Whenever possible, the lower limbs should be abducted and supported at 90° to the hips, and 90° at the knees and ankles. A pommel may be necessary to maintain abduction. Prevention of external rotation of the hip will help to decrease the possibility of inversion occurring at the ankles.

Weight should be taken equally through both feet and the foot-plate should be adjusted, possibly by the use of wedges, to enable this to happen. Weight taken through the balls of the feet only, as when plantar flexion occurs, will increase any abnormal tone, and should be avoided if possible. Straps at 45° to the ankles may encourage weight bearing through the heels instead of through the balls of the feet. However, any strapping should be used with caution, and regularly checked and reviewed, in order that it does not increase abnormal tone, restrict circulation, or cause breakdown of the skin.

Trunk

Trunk alignment will follow good positioning of the hips. Lumbar supports, waist supports or a chest strap may be required to maintain this position. The amount of support required will depend on the patient's awareness and degree of independent control, as well as whether the emphasis is on preventing or correcting a deformity.

Upper limbs

The arms and hands need to be in a good position in order to reduce any abnormal patterning that may be in evidence, as well as to bring them within the field of vision and place them in a position where spontaneous interaction with the environment is possible.

To position the upper limbs out of a flexor pattern, the shoulders need to be protracted, slightly flexed and in external rotation, with elbows, wrist and fingers extended, and thumb abducted.

Both shoulders should be maintained at the same height so as not to disturb the alignment of the body.

Head

Head alignment is generally difficult to maintain, and a head rest, with a strap, may be necessary. Reclining the chair slightly may help to retain the head in the mid line. However, this may also increase extensor tone. Caution should be practised in cases of severe flexor tone in the neck, as restraining may increase this further. Soft collars are used by some in maintaining head control, but the author is not in favour of these, believing that such appliances may affect swallowing, cause rubbing, and increase flexor tone in the neck.

Other practical considerations

It is worth noting here that, if a patient has been carefully positioned, according to his individual needs, then this should be maintained by all. If other members of the treatment team are dissatisfied with the position the patient is in, believing it to promote pain and postural difficulties, or inhibit voluntary movement, they should confer with those responsible for positioning, and not alter this themselves. It is most disheartening to carefully position a patient, only to find that someone, with the best of intentions, has added a pillow here, or a bit of padding there, in order to make the patient 'more comfortable'. Adjusting the position in this manner may increase muscle tone, facilitate abnormal movement patterns, increase pain, and/or cause skin breakdown.

Once a good position has been achieved, all staff should be instructed in the importance of maintaining this, and in techniques of moving the patient from one position to another. A wall-chart or check-list will help those concerned with the daily care of the patient. It is important that the patient be moved with the minimum of handling, and with confidence, so that he is able to relax quickly in his new position. Noxious stimuli, as can be inadvertently administered in the process of transferring, will cause an increase in abnormal tone.

The requirements of the patient will constantly change and, therefore, the position should be reviewed daily. One does not want the patient to become dependent on the support provided, or encourage contractures, abnormal positioning, and skin breakdown. As the patient improves, less physical support should be provided during treatment sessions in order to encourage greater control of parts of the body, but care should be taken not to overtire the patient.

Attention must be paid to the condition of the skin in all patients who are unable to move independently due to either decreased awareness or motor impairment. For those patients who are restless or agitated, the carers should inspect the skin for signs of breakdown due to constant rubbing or knocking of limbs against parts of the chair (or bed), or against bony prominences. Care also needs to be taken with those who have impaired sensation.

Once the patient is sitting in a good position, care should be taken to place the chair in a visually interesting position, not facing the wall or excluding him/her from any group.

SPASTICITY

Spasticity is probably the most common physical disorder seen following head injury. It is characterized by hyperreflexia, hypertonia, and clonus. Hyperreflexia is seen as brisk and irradiating tendon jerks or phasic stretch reflex; hypertonia is an increased resistance to rapid passive stretch; and clonus is a series of repetitive muscle contractions elicited by a rapidly applied, but maintained, stretch (Chapman and Wiesendanger, 1982).

Following severe head injury, we may see abnormal tone ranging from minimal to severe in isolated muscles or muscle groups, affecting one side of the body, affecting all four limbs, head or trunk, or any combination of these. Frequently, spasticity occurs in combined flexor and extensor patterns, thus adding to the difficulty of inhibiting it.

Initially, the patterning of abnormal tone may regularly vary and the therapist should be continually alert to the changing needs of the patient, particularly in positioning to inhibit spasticity. It is not uncommon to find that, as motor recover occurs, the spasticity spontaneously subsides to a point where no treatment is necessary. In those patients who require treatment, the natural course of recovery is generally from proximal to distal, from mass to patterned, and from gross to isolated movement. However, the recovery process can stop at any point and it is unusual for the patient to regain full function.

Factors which will increase spasticity, and should therefore be avoided, include production of effort, poor body positioning, noxious stimuli, pain, fear and anxiety, weight of bed clothes on the body, pressure on the balls of the feet, and infections such as colds.

Deliberate stimulation, as recommended in Chapter 2, may

increase spasticity if present. It is, therefore, necessary for the therapist to be sensible in his/her approach, decide the order in which to meet the patient's needs, and, after application of noxious stimuli, finish each session with an activity which will relax the patient, and reposition the patient in order to inhibit the spasticity. As the patient becomes more aware, activities which encourage, or reinforce, abnormal tone should be avoided.

Treatment approaches

There are several methods of treatment used for the control of spasticity, and the treatment team as a whole should decide on the best approach, or combination of approaches, for each patient. Factors which may influence the decision include: age of the patient, ability of the patient to co-operate, severity and combination of spasticity, associated physical disorders and ability and preferences of individual members of the treatment team.

Good positioning of the body is valuable in inhibiting the spasticity, as already discussed, and provides a firm base from which movements can be facilitated. All staff should diligently ensure that the recommended positions are strictly adhered to, whilst the physiotherapist and/or occupational therapist will use techniques to facilitate normal movement patterns.

The dynamic approach to inhibiting spasticity and facilitating movement are well known by the practising clinician, and many good textbooks are available. However, the following are a selection of alternative approaches which could be considered by the treatment team, to be used in conjunction with standard techniques, particularly in difficult cases.

Splinting

Plaster casts and other sorts of splints have been used very effectively in both the upper and lower extremities to reduce spasticity, prevent contractures and to increase range of movement. However, the popularity of orthoses is varied, with some therapists never using splinting and others always doing so (Neuhaus *et al.*, 1981).

Many people over the years have recommended the use of splints for reducing spasticity in upper and lower limbs (for example Brennon, 1959; Kaplan, 1962; Snook, 1979; King, 1982; McPherson *et al.*, 1982). The discussions go on as to the benefits of volar versus

Figure 5.1 Thermoplastic wedges being used to maintain the fingers in abduction. The volar splint, which can reduce spasticity, prevent contractures and increase the range of movement, should be worn following a timetable of approximately two–four hours on/two–four hours off.

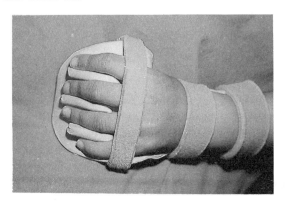

dorsal, part-time versus full-time, full stretch versus no stretch and temporary versus permanent benefits. Whatever the arguments for or against splinting, it is inevitable that some patients with moderate to severe spasticity cannot be managed by positioning and movement facilitation alone. This may be due not only to the severity of spasticity, but also to lack of the patient's co-operation caused by decreased level of awareness or disorders of behaviour.

The hand: the orthosis for the wrist/hand/finger, favoured by the author, is that recommended by Peterson (1985), in which the hand is splinted in a position where neither the extensor muscles nor the flexor muscles are in full stretch. This volar splint can be fabricated in an unlined thermoplastic material which takes up the contours of the hand easily. To aid fabrication of the orthosis, the patient must be positioned so that the palmar surface is accessible, and this can be achieved by lying the patient supine so that the palm is face up, or with the patient sitting (if she/he is able to) with his hand behind his/her back.

In order to determine the joint positions for splinting, the range of movement of the joints distal to the elbow are estimated by passively extending the parts: wrist extension is then decreased by 10°. The proximal interphalangeal joints and metacarpo-phalangeal joints should be placed at an angle as near to 45° as possible, and the thumb should be placed in opposition. The fingers should be abducted, and can be held in abduction by leather loops or by thermoplastic bridges between them (see Figure 5.1). The splint can be held in place by straps at the proximal edge, wrist and over the proximal phalanges. A timetable of approximately two to four hours on and two to four hours off, although not recommended by Peterson, should be used because prolonged wearing may increase tone, pain, stiffness of joints and/or maceration of tissue.

Staff, relatives and patients can be taught to put the splint on and take it off in order to clean the splint and skin, exercise the upper limb, and check for rubbing. Great care should be taken to prevent breakdown of the skin by ill-fitting splints because pain will increase the tone that you are trying to decrease. Care should also be taken in checking for rubbing of skin on other parts of the body, such as the chest.

This splint is a serial splint, and as the spasticity reduces and the range of motion becomes greater the splint should be remoulded (see

Figure 5.2 Wrist/hand/finger orthosis used to reduce flexor spasticity (the effect is throughout the whole of the upper limb): (a) the first splint in the series; (b) the last splint six weeks later.

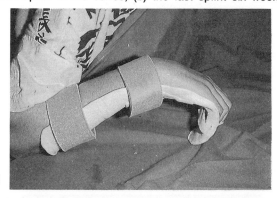

(a)

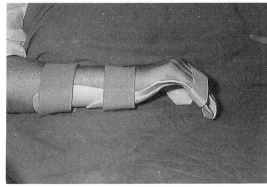

(b)

Figure 5.2). Generally this can be done every two to three days. In the author's experience, success with this splint has generally been seen in those who respond to ice as a method of reducing spasticity.

The elbow: increased tone in the flexors of the elbow can be reduced by using a flexor stop which can be adjusted as the range of motion increases (King, 1982). King originally recommended the use of a plaster cast around the upper arm with an outlying flexor stop which maintained the elbow in its maximum extension (which could be gained through gentle, passive stretch), but allowed extension to occur as the spasticity decreased. When the elbow could move 10° out of the splint, the splint was changed to, again, hold the limb in full extension (see Figure 5.3).

Figure 5.3 An orthosis for reducing spasticity in the elbow. The orthosis has a thermoplastic cuff around the upper arm with a flexor stop outrigger.

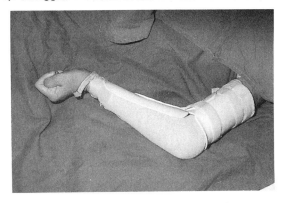

Thermoplastic material can be used instead of plaster; it has the advantage of being lighter and easier to reshape and clean. The upper arm segment can be made up of two shells which can be clamped together and held securely with Velcro.

Once the elbow has reached full extension minus 15°, the splint can be removed and worn at night only for maintenance purposes.

In order to fabricate splints without causing excessive fear, and therefore increasing spasticity, the patient should be carefully prepared for this session. Relaxation techniques should be practised, and peace and calm maintained throughout the process. Avoiding associated reactions and directing the patient's attention elsewhere is advised.

Plaster casting: this is an effective means of preventing and correcting contractures, particularly of the ankle, knee, and elbow, but such casts require regular changing and inspection.

Air splints: orally inflated splints can be fitted to a spastic limb and inflated to conform to and support it. Johnston (1984), believes that air splints can be used for two purposes: to re-educated sensory discrimination by the sustained pressure it exerts over the limb; and to inhibit muscle spasm by holding the limb in an anti-spasm pattern. Johnston recommends the use of splints for two periods of one hour daily, whilst under supervision, and for each period to be immediately followed by exercise. Exercise can be performed whilst in air splints as they give the extremity the stability needed to aid exercise to specific body parts, for example the shoulder.

The air splint can also be used to aid weight-bearing through an affected limb; enabling this to be carried out much earlier and much more intensively than is otherwise possible.

Many other techniques are available to the clinician for the prevention and correction of spasticity, and there is a need to identify those which are going to be effective on the individual patient. The maintenance of reduced spasticity should also be given considerable attention. Again, one must be flexible in one's approach, be sensitive to changing needs, and approach the problem as a team, aware of the expertise of colleagues.

ATAXIA

Ataxia is a disturbance of voluntary movement seen as a marked lack of co-ordination of movement. A patient may have minimum to severe ataxia of the total body, trunk or upper or lower extremities, and this may be temporary to permanent following head injury.

Adding weights can be an effective way of controlling a tremor during activity, but this will not decrease the ataxia. The point of origin (body part) of the tremor should be carefully assessed and this will indicate the correct placement for the weights. The amount of weight applied will depend on the area to which it is applied, and the size and age of the patient. The weights should be added gradually in order to accustom the patient to carrying an extra load.

Careful assessment will also indicate compensatory techniques which may be employed by the patient. For example, if one anchors an affected body part, as in leaning an elbow on a table, one will be required to co-ordinate only the parts of the body distal to the anchor point when carrying out an activity (Turner, 1981).

Patients will benefit from slowing activities down to a pace where the tremor can be controlled. For training, design exercises which incorporate purposeful activity, and which require the patient to move objects from one area to another (for example use wooden noughts-and-crosses or large draughts).

SENSORY IMPAIRMENT

Sensory impairment, if present, may range from partial to total loss, and usually affects the higher discriminatory function rather than the primary sensations, for example the patient may feel touch but be unable to localize it, and may feel the difference between hot and cold but be unable to distinguish the temperature in between (Bobath, 1977).

Sensory extinction

Tactile extinction is a failure to identify a stimulus to an affected part when at the same time the same stimulus is applied to the corresponding part of the body, although the stimulus would be identified if applied on its own to the affected side of the body (see Chapter 4).

Stereognosis

Stereognosis is the ability to identify an object by feel, and this may be defective following severe head-injury. When the patient is alert and able to follow instructions, test by occluding the patient's vision (covering the hand rather than covering the eyes) and asking him/her to identify small objects by feeling them. Caution should be practised because objects can be identified by the noise they make if they bang against a table or other hard surface.

Proprioception

Proprioception is the sense of position and movement as determined by receptors located in the deep tissue of muscles, tendons, periosteum and joints (Eggars, 1983). Without sufficient feedback on position and movement, the patient will not know how to move and this may cause disuse of a limb even if the motor power is good.

Proprioception can be treated for by occluding the patient's vision and moving his/her fingers, or toes, one at a time, randomly up or down (but not to the extent that pain or stretch reflex is elicited), and asking the patient to indicate the direction and the degree of movement. The finger or toe being moved should not touch other fingers or toes during testing, nor should the patient's fingers be allowed to touch the palm of his/her hand.

If the patient is unable to identify the direction of movement in smaller joints, then the larger joints should be tested. If the patient is unable to respond verbally, she/he may be able to indicate the direction of movement by demonstrating with the other hand or foot, if body schema is intact. If it is necessary to support the limb during testing, for example when working on the elbow or wrist, the support given should be light, as information received from pressure on the flexors or extensors may aid identification of movement.

Where abnormal proprioception exists, the therapist should incorporate into his/her treatment programme activities designed to improve proprioceptive feedback. Initially these should include passive movement of the affected joints so the patient can identify the sensations received; this should be done with the patient watching. The next stage is for the patient to move his/her affected joints, with the unaffected arm, again whilst watching.

To progress, the patient must start to carry out purposeful activity involving the affected joints aided by an unaffected part, for example bilateral draughts. Adding different weights, incorporating change of direction, giving resistance to movement, and weight bearing through an affected limb will provide stimulation for the proprioceptors.

Air splints can also be used to re-establish deep sensations, particularly in conjunction with a mechanical intermittent pressure pump (Johnston, 1984). However, great care needs to be taken in using such an aid, and careful assessment of the degree of spasticity and amount of sensory loss is recommended. It is also recommended that the intermittent pressure programme is used only in conjunction with a sustained pressure programme (see the section on spasticity).

Implications

Sensory impairment has implications for rehabilitation in that it can lead to neglect of parts of the body; this, in turn, may be significant in terms of the patient's ability to manipulate tools. Sensory impairment may also lead to injury of parts of the body because the patient may not recognize when she/he is at risk from hazards such as burning or overstretching weak muscles.

MUSCULAR WEAKNESS OR PARALYSIS

Muscular weakness or paralysis may be seen following head injury and it may affect any part of the body, or a combination of parts. This impairment may abate as the patient recovers, it may be permanent or it may develop into spasticity.

Where motor weakness or paralysis is apparent, the therapist must maintain the range of movement as well as prevent contractures which may lead to further loss of function and increased pain. If sensory loss accompanies weakness, efforts should be made to make the patient continually aware of the affected part, by positioning the part within the patient's visual field, and by training him/her to take responsibility for that part.

The physiotherapist, working with the occupational therapist, will be able to guide members of the treatment team through the necessary patterns of passive movements indicated, instruct on the precautions to take in daily care activities (particularly involving the shoulder joint), and instruct in appropriate techniques for moving the patient from one position or location to another in order to prevent the reinforcement of abnormal movement patterns, or damage to physical structures.

A patient who is able and willing to co-operate in treatment activities, can be taught to self-range affected joints. We must be aware that patients can quickly adopt a one-handed method of working, causing disuse of the affected side, and therefore wide bilateral activities are essential in bringing the affected extremity into function. When activities only require a one-handed approach, the patient should bear weight through the affected side in order to stimulate the proprioceptors.

It is up to all team members to ensure the patient adopts good positions and that she/he accepts responsibility for her/his affected extremity or extremities. It is also the responsibility of the treatment team members to prevent damage to affected joints, such as subluxation of the shoulder, and this can be done by education of staff, relatives, and the patient, and by regular reviewing of the patient's needs.

RANGE OF MOVEMENT

Range of motion may be limited by contractures of soft tissue, tendon shortening, additional bony injuries, increased muscle tone, or by heterotopic ossification. Decorticate or decerebrate rigidity, in the initial phase, will indicate possible restricted range of motion as recovery occurs. Range of motion can be assessed by passive movement of the joints.

If range of motion is restricted, investigations should be made in order to determine the exact nature of the problem. It should be the responsibility of all members of the treatment team to draw to the attention of the medical staff, and others, any problems encountered so that they can be investigated.

Depending on the cause of reduced range of motion, further loss of range should be prevented, usually by passive movement of joints and maintaining a good position. Serial splinting can sometimes increase range, particularly with contractures of soft tissue.

VISUAL DISORDERS

Apart from disorders of visual perception, for example in interpreting what is seen, the patient may experience defective vision following head injury, including visual field defects, double vision (diplopia), nystagmus (unco-ordinated movements of the eyes), and blindness.

Visual field defects are caused by interruption of the visual pathways; the point at which the pathways are interrupted determines the field of dysfunction. Visual field defects include homonymous hemianopia (loss of the left or the right half of the visual field in each eye), upper or lower homonymous quadrants, and blindness in one or both eyes.

It is important for the therapist to determine early in the recovery stage if visual disorders exist, and, if so, whether they have a physical basis or are perceptual in nature. It is not always apparent that the patient has a disorder of vision, particularly in those who readily compensate without prompting. However, if suspected, special investigations should be requested.

If the disorder has a physical basis, compensatory tactics can be employed which will hopefully reduce frustration. The patient should be taught scanning techniques, and efforts should be made, initially, to bring necessary items, tasks or information, within the existing visual field. If the patient experiences double vision, an eye-patch will help to alleviate this, although she/he may find it uncomfortable or irritating to wear it and therefore refuse to do so. If an eye-patch is used, it should be worn equally by the two eyes.

Nystagmus may also be helped with an eye-patch – the patch reduces the need to co-ordinate visual input.

HEARING

We rely heavily on the ability to communicate verbally, and this requires the ability to produce both meaningful speech, and to hear, interpret, and respond to what we hear. Initially, it should be assumed that the patient can hear until proven otherwise. Later, if there is a difficulty in communication, it can be incorrectly assumed that hearing is intact but that there is some disorder in auditory perception or attentional ability.

We generally give more visual and tactile cues in communication than we believe and so it is possible that a patient will function, albeit in a disorientated and confused manner, with a hearing deficit. It is therefore easy to overlook defective hearing in patients who are thought to be functioning at a reduced level.

Hearing loss can be of a temporary nature, caused by a torn eardrum, blood in the middle ear, or a fractured temporal bone. Damage can, however, be more permanent. If it is considered that the patient has hearing difficulties, whatever the degree, she/he should be referred for investigations. In order to avoid increasing the patient's confusion and frustration, efforts should be made by the team to ensure that communication, in cases of defective hearing, is channelled through other sensory receptors.

It should be remembered that some patients may be able to hear, but not be able to interpret what they are hearing, for example a patient may be able to hear water running, but not be able to identify the sound. In cases of auditory perceptual disorders, as in other receptive disorders of language, patients should be referred to the speech therapist for assessment and treatment. The speech therapist will be able to advise on strategies to adopt in order to help the patient cope with auditory dysfunction. If the speech therapist is unable to see the patient regularly for treatment, she/he will be able to provide a programme of therapeutic exercises which any member of the treatment team, or a relative, can work on with the patient.

Initially, the patient may be very sensitive to noise, and, therefore, should be very gradually accustomed to coping with greater noise levels. Working with the patient in an environment which is too noisy will defeat the objectives of any treatment session because she/he will be unable to pay attention to any activity. This may be a permanent problem.

SPEECH

Apart from the thought processes which lead to speech, the physical ability to speak may be impaired following head injury. Dysarthria, caused by nerve impairment, is a partial or complete inability to co-ordinate the muscles involved in the production of speech.

The speech therapist will be able to identify area(s) of difficulty and the treatment(s) required. It is essential that when such difficulties exist a consistent approach is adopted by all in order to promote good communication, to prevent frustration on the part of the patient and/or others, to prevent the patient adopting bad speech habits and to prevent further loss of function.

If the speech therapist is able to visit the patient only once a week she/he should be able to provide exercises for the patient to follow under the guidance of either a relative or member of staff. For this to be effective, communication between the speech therapist and assigned co-workers needs to be regular and consistent.

EPILEPSY

Epilepsy, in one form or another, may occur following severe head injury, with about 5% of patients having a first fit within a week (early onset), and about 5% developing late traumatic epilepsy (more than seven days after injury). In those patients developing late traumatic epilepsy, the incidence will be greater in relation to length of coma, (Jennet, 1983; Guidice and Berchou, 1987).

Of those patients who experience the first fit within the first week of injury, it is estimated that only 25% will also experience late traumatic epilepsy. Although late onset is classified as starting more than seven days post injury it can take years before onset.

The type of fit will vary considerably from patient to patient and will range from *grand mal* to minor fits which may go unnoticed, such as fits which may only, for example, cause a temporary break in concentration/attention. The therapist working with the patient should always be alert to the possibility of fits and report anything that she/he considers to be indicative of epilepsy. Staff should also be familiar with safe procedures to adopt following an epileptic fit.

If late traumatic epilepsy develops, education of the patient and the relatives is important if they are to understand its management. In certain cases, it may be appropriate to make contact with the British Epilepsy Association, for help, guidance, and support.

PROTECTIVE HELMETS

In cases where there has been removal of a bone flap covering the brain, external protection may be needed. Patients requiring it include those who are restless and agitated, and, perhaps, prone to wandering; those who are anxious regarding lack of bony protection (and are reluctant to comply with treatment as a result); and patients who are involved in a vigorous physical programme. Relatives and staff may also feel more confident handling patients who have sufficient protection against sustaining further injury to the brain. Considering each patient on his/her individual needs, protection may be indicated only for sessions in physiotherapy, during other physical activity, or for periods outside the hospital when walking over rough ground or in crowds.

If it is anticipated that a cranioplasty will not be performed for some time, if at all, and if the team have decided that a helmet is indicated, a request should be made to the surgical fitters within the hospital for the fabrication of a sturdy helmet. If temporary protection is required, a helmet can be fabricated easily by the occupational therapist or a physiotherapist who is experienced in the making of splints.

For the fabrication of a temporary helmet, the therapist will require a minimum supply of thermoplastic material, self-adhesive lining felt, Velcro, and leather. The process is as follows:

1. Measure the circumference of the head, from base of the skull around the forehead (measurement 'A').
2. Cut out a strip of thermoplastic material the length of measurement 'A' plus 1 in, and approximately 1 in wide. Line this piece with self-adhesive felt.
3. Depending on the material used, put a thin protective covering over the head. Heat the material to the correct moulding temperature, and mould around the head, from base of the skull

Figure 5.4 The thermoplastic strip around the circumference of the head (base of neck to forehead) provides the foundation of the helmet.

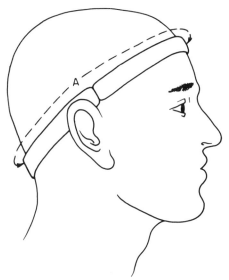

to the forehead. The opening should be formed by the butting of the edges and should be placed directly opposite the area of bone loss. Secure with a bandage until firm (hardening time is dependent on material used). Remove the bandage and secure the closure by firmly attaching self-adhesive Velcro straps (see Figure 5.4).

4. Measure from rim to rim, over the head, horizontal to the opening (measurement 'B'). Cut out a piece of self-adhesive felt the length of 'B' and 1 in wide. Cut out a piece of thermoplastic material the length of 'B' plus 2 in and 1 in wide. Attach the self-adhesive felt centrally on the thermoplastic strip.

5. Heat this strip to the required moulding temperature and mould centrally over the head, horizontal to the opening. Bond both ends of strip 'B' to strip 'A'. Allow the strip to harden (see Figure 5.5).

6. With the helmet skeleton still in place, make a template to cover the area of bone loss (measurement 'C'), extending to cover strip 'B' and the appropriate half-circumference of strip 'A'. Using the template, cut a piece of thermoplastic material to shape. Over the area of bone loss, place a piece of padding approximately ½ in to 1 in thick; this will be removed after moulding. Heat up the

Figure 5.5 The skeleton of the temporary helmet.

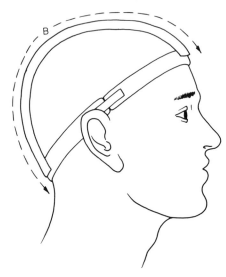

Figure 5.6 The helmet skeleton with the area of bone loss covered with thermoplastic material.

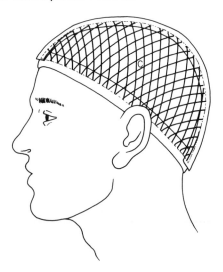

thermoplastic and mould over the padding, bonding the edges securely to strips 'A' and 'B'. Allow to set. Caution should be practised in preventing any pressure being placed over the area of bone loss (see Figure 5.6).

7. Remove the helmet and the last padding applied. Inspect the skin for pressure areas and make fine adjustments to the fit if these are present. Ensure that no rough edges are present and that the joints are securely bonded.

8. At this point, it must be considered if the helmet is rigid enough for protection. If not, carefully positioned, rigid piece(s) of thermoplastic material can be applied. Care should be taken not to make the helmet unsightly.

9. Place the helmet back on the head of the patient and measure for the straps (measurement 'D'); a chin cup should be favoured as this clears the straps from around the throat. Fabricate and securely attach the straps. The straps need to be attached to the helmet at a point which will allow maximum stability and comfort. The type of fastenings used are subject to individual preference, however Velcro is very easy to apply. Velcro is also easy to undo and should not be used if the patient is liable to remove the helmet at inopportune moments (see Figure 5.7).

Figure 5.7 The complete temporary helmet with Velcro fastening straps and chin cup.

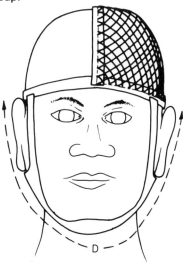

10. It is recommended that the helmet is labelled unobtrusively with the patient' name; the back and front should also be marked. Instructions should be given, and supported by an instruction sheet by the bed, about when the helmet should and should not be worn.

11. After fabrication, do not store the helmet anywhere hot as this will soften, and therefore, distort it.

SUMMARY

Physical dysfunction following severe head injury can be extremely complex and can tax the most competent therapist. Initially, the signs and symptoms will change frequently and will need reviewing daily in order to maintain good positions, maintain a good range of movement, prevent contractures and decubitus ulcers.

Thorough assessment is essential to determine the presence and severity of physical dysfunction, and to exclude other causes of loss of function. Following careful assessment, the team should identify the treatment approaches to be adopted, and these should be regularly reviewed as the needs of the patient change. The physiotherapist should always be consulted regarding the prevention and correction of physical dysfunction, and should be instrumental in co-ordinating the approach of the individual members of the treatment team.

Good positioning is essential in order to prevent increase in spasticity, contractures, decubitus ulcers, and respiratory disorders. This may be difficult initially due to the presence of associated injuries and presence of abnormal tone, the use of support and monitoring systems, and the patient's decreased level of consciousness.

The position in the bed or chair once determined, should be strictly maintained by all concerned, and regularly reviewed. The positions should be charted for the benefit of everyone. Not only is good positioning important, but also the method of moving the patient from one position or location to another; methods chosen should be practised by everyone.

Spasticity is one of the most common complications in head injury. Dynamic approaches to the reduction of spasticity are well known. However, with reduced co-operation from the patient these are often difficult to put into practice and therefore we may need to be more divergent in our thinking and select and combine different treatments. Splinting and casting of extremities should not be ruled out as a valid approach.

Ataxia, sensory impairment, muscle weakness or paralysis, and restricted range of joint motion may all be seen independently of each other, or in any combination. Associated injuries may add complications, as may medical conditions which affected the individual prior to, or as a consequence of, the injury.

If it is felt that the treatment team do not have the knowledge or expertise to cope with the difficulties presented, and if transfer to a specialized unit is impossible, every effort should be made to bring in specialists to advise on treatment. Physiotherapists, occupational therapists and speech therapists from specialist centres are generally very willing to come and advise staff on the rehabilitation of an individual head-injured patient.

The consequences of head injury do not always include physical dysfunction, and therefore some patients will only require the minimum of supervision and guidance through the early stages of recovery, particularly in the areas of balance, co-ordination, and increase in fatigue levels. If, however, the patient has few, if any, physical disorders, the treatment team should not be lulled into an early withdrawal of treatment or support; the psychosocial consequences can cause the most difficult problems following head injury.

6

Return to the community

Throughout this book, the importance of the role of the relative has been emphasized, as has the need to support the family who are at least as affected as the patient.

Support for the family should be automatic, and the process will help to build a rapport between staff and relatives. The therapist should continually be aware of the needs of the family in order to identify the level of support necessary. In many cases, the treatment team may identify a key worker to communicate with the family in order to prevent conflicting information from being given by different people. However, even if a key worker is elected, relatives should not be discouraged from communicating with other members of the treatment team unless this is seen as impeding the patient's progress.

THE SOCIAL WORKER

The social worker is a very important member of the treatment team who may be involved with the family, and the patient, from day 1 of injury. The social worker is employed by the local government but can be based in a variety of settings – for example community teams, health centres and hospitals. As with all team members, communication is vital if the patient is to benefit from the multi-professional approach.

During the immediate crisis stage, the social worker should be involved in the intensive care situation where life and death issues are unclear. As the outcome of injury becomes more apparent, and as it is seen that the patient is going to survive, the social worker will turn the focus of counselling onto disability awareness and acceptance.

During the early days, many practical issues exist which need the attention of the relatives or other relevant persons. For example, to allow the relatives to visit regularly, help may be needed to look after children or dependants, financial help may be required to support the family, and legal proceedings may need to be initiated. Many people are not aware of what they need to do in the event of serious injury to a relative, furthermore it is not the best time to cope with these issues, so help is needed to guide them through the practicalities.

The social worker is well equipped to offer practical help and guidance to the relatives, and, later, to the patient himself. The social worker will have the knowledge of where to seek help, will have the appropriate contacts, and will be aware of the legal rights of the individuals involved. She/he should also be responsible for the gathering of relevant information on the patient and family, and for the dissemination of this information to other members of the treatment team.

In many instances, if the social worker is able to give the intensive support required, she/he is ideally suited to taking the role of the key worker because involvement does not automatically cease at the time of discharge. The social worker is not generally involved directly in the treatment of the patient (although at a later stage may be involved in the process of counselling), and may be seen by relatives as set apart from the treatment team, and, therefore, in a better position to be the family's advocate at team meetings.

HOME VISITING

During the patient's stay in hospital, the relatives should be encouraged to take some responsibility, with support, for his/her care, and, therefore, should acquire confidence in handling and caring for the patient. The hospital is very different from home, in that it is a protected environment where professionals are readily available to take charge should any emergency arise, and help is at hand to lift, restrain and support. A relative can readily walk away from the hospital, should the situation become too difficult to handle or should she/he become too tired to cope with the patient. It is not to be suggested that this is an easy time for the carers, but the support systems are physically in evidence, as is the structure for responsibility, which is ultimately not that of the relatives.

As the patient becomes more alert and medically stable, a home visit should be considered, as long as the home situation is stable, the patient has a home to visit, the home is within easy access, and the relatives are assessed as being able to cope with this next stage.

The patients making a home visit must be able to attend to the environment and be medically stable, and it must be physically possible to transport him/her. Access to the home needs to be determined prior to arranging the visit and guidelines need to be given to the relatives as to the purpose of the exercise and the constraints, i.e. who should be there, who to dissuade from coming, timing. The family's expectations should be carefully explored.

A home visit at this stage is seen as part of the rehabilitation programme and *not* as a means of emptying hospital beds. It should be stressed to the relatives that no pressure is currently being placed upon them to take the patient home before she/he, or the family, is ready and able to cope.

Home visit guidelines

Determine objectives

These will be different for each patient. Staff should not be over-ambitious in what they want to achieve in one session; for many patients and relatives, just being together at home for the first time may be overwhelming. The objectives of a home visit include:

1. To return the patient to a familiar environment for the purposes of sensory stimulation.
2. To assess the responses, or coping mechanisms, of the family and patient within their own environment, for example without the security of the clinical setting, and to assess the level of support required.
3. To raise the morales of both patient and relative(s).
4. To assess the home situation with regard to future visits, escorted and unescorted, extensions to overnight stays, and, finally, discharge.
5. To assess for equipment and adaptations required in the short term, to enable further home visits of increasing duration, and overnight stays, to be planned.
6. To gather information for long-term planning.

Determine timing of the first visit

This will be dependent on:

1. Stable medical condition, as determined by the consultant in charge. The state should be such that the patient can be moved from a safe environment, and therefore, away from support systems.
2. Patient's awareness of the environment and changes within this.
3. Ability of the relatives to cope with the stresses created by a home visit.
4. Access to appropriate transportation.
5. Availability of appropriate support staff to accompany the patient on a home visit.
6. The duration of visit will be determined to a great extent by the tolerance of the patient.

Determine transport required

The type of transport required will be dependent on:

1. Physical state of the patient; amount of support required; size of the patient; ability to transfer from chair to car to chair; additional injuries.
2. Behaviour exhibited by the patient.
3. Transport available: staff car, taxi, hospital ambulance with or without tail-lift. If a staff member is using his/her own car, this should be done only with adequate insurance cover for such activities.
4. Number of attendants required, remembering that fewer staff are less imposing.
5. Type and amount of equipment required, for example wheelchair, walking aid.
6. Distance between home and hospital.

Determine escorts required

The number or type of escorts required will be dependent on:

1. The physical needs of the patient, for instance the patient may require the attendance of a nurse if a specific medical problem is identified.

97

2. The expertise, ability and experience of individual members of the treatment team.
3. Intensity of rapport between an individual member of the treatment team and the relatives and/or patient; this may be a key worker or another person with whom the patient identifies strongly.
4. Specific objectives may determine the presence of a certain professional representative, for example the need to assess for equipment and adaptations means that an occupational therapist should be present.
5. It is not recommended that less than two members of staff attend the home visit, for reasons of safety of both patient and staff. However, too many escorts will be intrusive.
6. It may be appropriate to meet professionals from other agencies at the home. For example, if equipment and adaptations are going to be required, it is appropriate for a community occupational therapist to attend as this will give him/her the opportunity to meet the patient in his/her own home, as well as to assess the requirements in conjunction with those who are aware of present abilities and prognosis.

Identify barriers

There may be physical barriers to conducting an effective home visit and these need to be identified either by a preliminary visit by staff only or by enquiry. Physical problems include:

1. Access may be via stairs or steep steps or there may be insufficient turning areas for a wheelchair at access points.
2. Basic facilities, such as the lavatory, may cause problems so it may be necessary to take specific equipment to the home.
3. The periods during the day when the patient is least co-operative or alert should be avoided when planning the home visit.
4. Feed and medication times should be checked and avoided for the home visit.

Preparation

Adequate preparation for the home visit is essential if it is to be successful; this should include:

1. Seeking written medical approval before commencing arrangements.

2. Seeking the permission of the relative(s), and/or patient if appropriate.
3. Communicating with the family on the objectives of the home visit, and exploring their expectations. This is a stressful exercise for the family as it will bring the consequences of the injury into reality. Support is essential at this time and should come from the treatment team, other family members, and friends.
4. Stressing to both the relatives and patient that the patient has to return to the hospital at the end of the visit.
5. Ensuring that the patient has suitable clothing to travel home in, taking into account seasonal variations. Special attention must be paid to footwear.
6. Confirming with the family the date and time (verbally and in writing), and confirming the exact location of the home. Give the relatives guidelines to follow, such as dissuading anyone other than the immediate family from visiting at that time, and leaving the house in its 'natural' state, as it would be remembered by the patient.
7. Careful co-ordination of transport is vital, ensuring that the times are confirmed for both departure from hospital to arrival at home and vice versa.
8. Notifying any staff who may be affected by the visit, for example the patient may have to miss a treatment session with another professional.
9. Identifying the equipment required and ensuring that staff are prepared for any eventuality. Equipment needed may include such items as a wheelchair or walking frame, incontinence pads, spare catheter bag, sick bowl and urinal. A note book, pen and tape-measure are essential, as is staff identification.
10. Checking out channels of communication between home and hospital, for example is there a telephone in the house; where is the nearest call box; does the department/hospital have a portable 'phone which can be taken; has the car/ambulance/taxi some means of communication and will they be waiting throughout the home visit?
11. Determining the role of each individual accompanying the patient: fact-finding, supportive, directive, observational.
12. Notifying the ward of the exact time of departure and return.

During the home visit

The form the home visit will take will be dictated by the objectives identified. However, the following should be taken into consideration:

1. If at all possible, the staff should be relatively unobtrusive and allow the relatives and patient some time alone. However, the staff should stay close enough at hand to know what is happening at all times, and to intervene if difficulties arise.
2. It is essential that the patient or relative(s) does not feel 'rushed' and the escorts may have to resign themselves to carrying out only a part of what they wished to achieve.
3. It should be remembered that the escorts are guests in the patient's home and can only suggest how the home visit should be conducted. However, if any activity embarked on by the patient is considered to be unsuitable, whether for health and safety reasons or other, the staff must use discretion and act accordingly. It is the duty of any professional to advise the patient of any serious risk of substantial harm.
4. If the therapist has any reservations about the ability of the patient or relative to carry out a specified activity, that part of the assessment/visit should be forfeited.
5. The escorts are in the home only with the express or implied consent of the occupier. If the consent is withdrawn the escorts then become trespassers, and the occupier can then take steps to remove them.
6. If a minor accident occurs when the patient is in the home, record the occurrence. This should be officially reported on return to the hospital.
7. For self-protection against charges of theft, no rooms should be entered unless accompanied by the patient or relative.

On return to the hospital

The home visit is not complete until the following have been carried out:

1. Make sure the patient is returned safely to the ward and made comfortable.
2. Give immediate feedback to the ward staff, making sure that all information relevant to the patient's immediate care is communicated. Make a hand-written entry in the patient's records confirming the information given to the nursing staff on return.

Feedback

The treatment team, including the relatives, will require feedback from this visit in order to aid treatment planning, and this should include:

1. A written report identifying existing facilities, patient's physical level of ability as demonstrated within the home, problem areas, patient's response to home situation, relatives' response, and, finally, recommendations regarding future home visits, rehabilitation requirements, and equipment and adaptations needed.
2. Verbal feedback to the treatment team for planning purposes.
3. Exploring the relatives' thoughts and feelings regarding the exercise, and giving positive feedback and encouragement. The family may be in need of considerable support at this point in order to work through their expectations, as compared to the reality of the home visit.

FOLLOWING THE HOME VISIT

The home visit is seen as part of the preparation for a planned discharge, but should only be seen as *one* in a series of progressive visits. This should also be reinforced to the family in order for them to be comfortable with the concept of gradually taking more responsibility for the care of the patient.

The home visit(s) will highlight the consequences of the injury, with relatives seeing the patient in a familiar setting but without taking his/her usual role within the family. They may feel repelled by what they see, unable to cope with, for example, incontinence, dribbling, bad behaviour, changed personality, passive responses or lack of recognition for something which was once important. All these may seem much more acceptable within the sick role in hospital, and this will all need to be talked carefully through before the next stage is reached.

The next stage should involve the relatives taking the patient home on their own, for a short period of about one hour, as long as no barriers have been identified to make this unrealistic. In order to achieve this the relatives must be confident in handling the patient in all areas of cleaning, changing clothes, toilet routines, transferring from chair to car and so on. The relatives must also be capable of any special procedures which the patient requires, for example, in order to maintain a high fluid intake.

It may be felt that further home visits require the support of a staff member, in order to train the relatives within the confines of their own home, or in order to increase confidence. Every effort should be made to provide this support.

Home visits should progress, ideally, from a one-hour visit, to a two-hour visit, to a meal-time visit, to an overnight stay, to a weekend stay and so on. The home visits require careful monitoring at all stages in order to prevent problems. The stages should not be moved through too quickly, even though it is felt that the family can cope, because community re-entry requires a considerable amount of adaptation by both parties.

It is also worth noting that following each home visit, a response from the patient can be expected, and that may range from being elated, to being depressed and unco-operative on return to the hospital. The patient will need a lot of support at this point as he may not be able to understand why his liberty is being restricted by being kept in hospital, he may be frustrated by his poor function, may not understand the relevance of his rehabilitation programme, and may be feeling rejected by his family.

A RELATIVE'S EXPERIENCE

One wife writes of her experience at the time of the first escorted home visit, which was four months after the injury, and the first unescorted home visit:

8 August 1987

'Malc's O.T. put me on the spot today when she asked me if I would like to have Malc home for a visit. I didn't know what to say, it had been mentioned in the past but now Jackie was actually asking me. My first question was 'will you be there?' I was actually frightened of being alone with him, with no medical staff to help if I needed them. Malc still had a catheter so he would have to wear a leg-bag; everything seemed very complicated. He was also still in a wheelchair, which made getting into the house very difficult. Jackie told me not to worry. She said it would be very stimulating for Malc and she assured me that she and Ruth wouldn't leave the house.

A date was made for the following Tuesday.'

12 August 1987

'I didn't sleep a wink last night worrying about the visit. I got up really early and made cakes and cleaned the house from top to bottom. I wanted everything to be just so. It had been arranged that I go into the hospital and see the whole visit through. I arrived at the hospital at 1 p.m. and excitedly told Malc where he was going. I struggled to put a jogging suit on him. He had been constantly sliding out of the wheelchair, so I securely fastened him in. Jackie arrived and asked me if I was all right and I was quite happy in what I was doing; I said yes not knowing whether I was.

Jackie pushed Malc to the front entrance after a lot of cheers from the lads on the ward. We were met by Ruth who was to drive us home. For some unknown reason I thought he would travel in the back of the car, but after a great deal of effort he was lifted into the front. Travelling along the Hagley Road is some experience for anyone but Malc was just fascinated by the hustle and bustle of the traffic. When we finally pulled up outside our house his face was a picture: he beamed at the sight of home. He anxiously fumbled for the door handle to escape from the car. Neighbours poured out of the houses to greet him, but I shall never forget the total look of shock on their faces. Getting the wheelchair into the house was extremely difficult because of the number of steps. We finally managed it and Malc was transferred to an armchair.

Mom had been caring for the children so she immediately left and Ruth and Jackie sat in another room. I couldn't believe that Malc was actually home, it hadn't been the way that I had expected it or wanted it, but he was here and he definitely knew it. Chris was very excited about his daddy coming home and he constantly fetched his toys to show him. I wanted everything to be as normal as possible so I switched on the television like Malc used to do. I then went to wake up Grace and I put her on Malc's lap; he stroked her tiny hand.

Malc always drank a lot of coffee so I rushed out to make him some. I gave it to him in a mug and he surprised me by drinking the whole lot. We had been having trouble giving him the tiniest sip in hospital. We ate cakes and I sat with my arms around him, it was perfect.

All too soon it was time for him to go back, it had been a great success, I only hope it will spark something off in his brain to make him fight harder.'

13 August 1987

'I was really pleased with the way things had gone yesterday, I felt as though we had achieved something and I knew Malc had had a great time. I walked into the ward all smiles this morning and I couldn't wait to talk to Malc about it all.

What a sight met my eyes, Malc was slumped in a chair, his head hung low and he was completely listless. I immediately thought he was ill. Dave was kneeling beside him to try and get him to drink some coffee. I just couldn't believe the difference in him, I had left him the previous evening on a real high.

I asked Dave what was wrong with him. He said he and some of the other nurses thought that Malc was very depressed at being brought back to the hospital. Dave told me that Malc was refusing to eat and drink and just wouldn't have anything to do with anyone. He told me to talk to him and try to explain that he had to come back. Dave the drew the curtains and left us alone. I told Malc that I desperately wanted him at home but at the moment I just couldn't manage, I told him that I had the children to care for and it just wouldn't be fair on anyone. I told him to fight and to do it harder than he had ever done and then he would be able to come home.

Malc wouldn't even look at me, he blamed me for taking him back and he was convinced that I didn't want him. My pity turned to anger and I told him to stop feeling sorry for himself because it would get him nowhere and least of all home. I then left in tears.

As the day went on I began to feel more and more guilty about what I had said to him, so I decided to take the children in and cheer him up. Chris took a bunch of flowers and Grace took some chocolates, Malc didn't exactly manage a smile but I think it perked him up a little.'

18 August 1987

'Malc came home for a few hours and I was left to cope alone.

He arrived at 11.45 a.m. with Ruth and Jackie; both came in for a little while to settle him down. I was extremely nervous about being left alone with him, but Ruth said that they were only at the end of a 'phone if I needed them. Ruth and Jackie then left and the house was left in complete silence.

Here I was alone with a baby, a toddler and a brain-damaged husband. I shut the thought out of my head and told myself to get on with it. I went on to prepare lunch – Malc's favourite, which is sweet-and-sour chicken. When lunch was ready I struggled to put Malc into his wheelchair. As I stood him up Malc was absolutely soaking. He hadn't got a catheter now, but he had a horrible sheath fitted onto him with a tube attached to it which led down to a leg bag. I ran to fetch soapy water and clean clothes.

Now you really have to imagine this. I struggled to take off Malc's clothes and I had to support him at the same time whilst I washed him. Christopher and Grace both witnessed all of this, but I had no choice as I couldn't shut them out because I had no-one to care for them. The chair was soaking wet so I had to disinfect it and put it outside to dry. Our lunch was cold and I was in tears.

I came out of the kitchen and remember thinking "well Karen, crying isn't going to get you anywhere, don't be stupid and go and have lunch". I wheeled Malc to the dining room, however, the wheelchair wouldn't go under the table so I had to lift Malc once again. Finally the meal was eaten and a great deal of mess was made by Malc because of lack of co-ordination. After lunch I put the children to bed and we went to watch T.V., it was lovely to be alone with him, but it wasn't my husband who I was left alone with, it was the mould of Malc but nothing more.

By the time Ruth and Jackie returned I was shattered, I had chronic backache through lifting him and I wanted to be left alone.'

DISCHARGE

No matter how much work you put into preparing the relatives for the patient's discharge, it is almost certain that they will never be ready. No matter how many home visits are conducted, or how well trained the relatives are in patient care, or how well supported, once discharge has taken place there is no going back and the final responsibility for care is placed on the relative's shoulders; or, at least, that is how it must feel.

Timing

The treatment team must continually review the patient's progress, and the relatives' ability to cope with the successive home visits. How many home visits are conducted, and to what extent, is determined according to both the patient's and the relatives' needs. In some cases, it may be felt that after an overnight stay all relevant parties feel confident enough to cope with discharge. With others, home visits may need to be taken to the extreme with several weekend visits taking place. For some, discharge to home may never be realistic.

Discharge, ideally, should be from inpatient care to daily out-patient treatment, within the same unit initially to ensure continuity of care. The timing of the discharge is important in that this should not coincide with periods where help cannot be sought from the treatment team if needed, or when essential services are not available, for example over bank holidays. Going home for weekends and nights is quite sufficient for most carers initially, particularly if the patient is highly dependent, and day care provision will help them to recharge batteries and spend time on themselves. If discharge is to be successful (not leading to early readmission), the carers must be given the opportunity to have regular breaks, resume some of their interests, spend time on or with other family members, and have the opportunity regularly to review the situation.

Provision of equipment and adaptations to the home

Discharge should not take place until the equipment and adaptations required to enable the patient to function as independently as possible, and to enable the relatives to take over physical care, have been provided. Apart from the practicalities of physical care, the home situation should be looked at with a view to the psychological aspects of living with an injured person, considering the personal space of the relatives and patient, and the degree of privacy that is required by those individuals.

Some relatives may resist having their home invaded by utilitarian pieces of equipment, or having their homes rearranged, for example bed and commode downstairs. The occupational therapist must work through this with them, exploring alternatives, as well as trying to identify the cause of the problem: this may be a way of delaying discharge if they feel that they cannot cope and do not feel able to say so.

The social services have a responsibility to provide disability equipment and adaptations. However, the need for these should, in the case of the head-injured person, be carefully assessed in terms of immediate and long-term requirements. The community occupational therapist is skilled in assessing for suitable equipment and adaptations, but will always look at alternative techniques to independence first; she/he should therefore be involved as early as possible in the management of discharge. It is possible to make the patient dependent by providing unnecessary equipment, or to restrict the patient's independence by providing too little. The use of any equipment provided should be regularly reviewed, as these may be easily discarded in the home in preference to some other technique which may need to be discouraged. The patient may also use equipment in a hospital setting because those in 'authority' tell him to, but he may not do so at the home.

As well as social services departments, equipment can be borrowed from nursing or home loan stores; in some areas the social services and health authority may work together so there are joint stores. Equipment may also be obtained from the occupational therapy department before discharge, either on short-term loan or for sale, or may be made to the patient's specifications. Wheelchairs are obtained on loan from the local disablement service centre (previously known as the artificial limb and appliance centre), and these are prescribed by a doctor, and assessed for by the occupational therapist or physiotherapist. Wheelchairs provided can be indoor/outdoor manual types or indoor assisted-propulsion types.

If equipment is needed in a hurry, and it is not available either from the social services or the health service, such organizations as the British Red Cross will hire certain items of equipment, for a small cost. All equipment, no matter where it is obtained, should be checked by the referring agent for its suitability, safe fitting, and correct use.

The potential for recovery does not always indicate the level of independence to be reached and therefore any negotiations in the early stages of rehabilitation for significant structural alterations should be approached cautiously. If structural alterations are eventually considered necessary, negotiations have to take place regarding the financing of the project, according to the nature of the tenancy, i.e. housing department if the home is owned by the local authority, housing association, or private. This will all take time and those concerned will have to exercise considerable patience if discharge has to be delayed until necessary alterations have been completed.

The fact that a patient has been referred for a specific piece of equipment, for adaptation to the home or for a community service, does not necessarily guarantee that it will be provided. One therefore has to look at the problem from all angles and recommend alternatives which may not be ideal, but will be practical.

Community services

Families may require community services in order to cope with the patient at home. Availability of community services will be dependent on the area of residence, but district nurses, home helps, laundry service, and voluntary agencies may be called upon to support the family and patient during trial leave, and at the time of, and following, discharge. As an out-patient, it may be possible for such services as bathing to be continued at the hospital, if these cannot be provided by the community, but these activities will neither be carried out in a 'normal' environment nor at the 'normal' time of day.

Before discharge, the treatment team, in consultation with the patient and his family, should identify the need for support in the community and this should be started at discharge, or alternative assistance identified and implemented. If a community service has been identified as necessary, hospital staff should ensure that it commences immediately and not several weeks later, leaving the family to struggle on alone.

Community services include:

1. *Bathing attendant*: request made by the general practitioner.
2. *District nurse*: for those who require nursing services for treatment of infections, pressure sores, bed-baths, help with getting into bed at night and getting out of bed in the morning, including help with dressing.
3. *Home helps*: help with a wide range of duties such as shopping, housework and preparing meals.
4. *Night watch/sitter service*: social services or private, depending on the area and availability. Will sit with the disabled person through the night in order to relieve the relatives who may be in need of rest.
5. *Carers groups*: such as the National Association of Carers. Some social services departments, health service districts and voluntary agencies run groups for carers to learn aspects of basic care of the disabled.
6. *Crossroads*: this is an organization in parts of the United Kingdom which offers help and support in aspects of care of the disabled person.

Other services exist, such as meals-on-wheels and day centre facilities, but the patient and relatives will not require these unless the hospital is unable to provide a continuation of the rehabilitation programme following inpatient discharge.

Allowances

It is important that financial benefits are considered, and applied for, prior to discharge. If the patient is thought to satisfy the criteria, it is crucial to apply for the government's attendance and mobility allowances. Invalid community care allowance for the relative, and the community care grant for the purposes of resettlement, should also not be forgotten.

Charities and trusts are very often useful sources of funding for specific items of equipment that the Department of Health will not provide, for example washing-machine or tumble-drier. Charities and trusts can also be a source of help with holidays through the Sick and Disabled Persons Act of 1970.

Practical training for the carers

Even if the relatives have been very active in the care of the head-injured patient in hospital, the need for further training may be apparent during the home visits. Training and practice may be needed in such tasks as getting the patient in and out of a car, manoeuvring a wheelchair around a tight corner or up steps, getting the patient in and out of a low bed, or on and off a lavatory in a tight space. Training will ensure that the handling is done with the minimum of fuss and with the minimum of risk of injury to either relative or patient. Much of this training can be done within the hospital in simulated conditions, as long as the therapist has collected accurate information regarding heights of existing equipment, floor space measurements and step heights. Equipment that is to be installed in the home can be practised on in the hospital under supervision.

However, it is not until you put this training into practice that you may find the difficulties. It is useful to work with the family in the home prior to discharge, thus giving the relative the opportunity to practise moving the patient from one position to another, from one room to another, and in and out of the house. Relatives must also be taught safety precautions, particularly in relation to their own circumstances. If the patient has reached a certain level of independence in self-care activities, working with the relatives and patient at home will give them confidence to continue to carry out these tasks. It is often much easier and quicker for the relative to help the patient to get dressed or washed, but they must be made to realize that it is better for the patient to do what she/he can independently. In pursuit of this, following discharge, it may be a good idea for some activities, such as dressing, to be continued at home under the supervision of a therapist, even though the patient may be attending the hospital daily.

SUPPORT GROUPS

Much of the support the family will receive from the different agencies will be of a physical nature and may, for many reasons, fall very short of providing emotional support. However, following discharge, the relatives soon begin to realize the full implications of head injury and it is at this point that help is needed.

Throughout Great Britain there is a network of support groups affiliated to Headway. These groups take different forms and shapes according to the needs of the members, some supporting head-injured victims, some the relatives of head-injured victims and some providing a combination of these. Relatives should be introduced to the local Headway group as early as possible in order to gain support from those who have been through the same experience.

Headway members can offer practical advice, will share experiences in order to help to solve problems, and will listen to those who need to just talk things over; to unburden oneself to someone who has been through the same experience is more helpful than talking to someone who cannot possibly imagine the significance of it all.

For staff working in areas where head-injured patients may be encountered, a knowledge of the local Headway group is useful and many professionals benefit enormously from attending. If insight is needed into family dynamics following head injury, and I suggest that it is essential, attending a Headway group is certainly the way to gain greater understanding, and therefore, empathy.

SUMMARY

The family is as affected, and in some ways more so, than the head-injured victim him/herself. It has been emphasized throughout this book that considerable support and understanding is needed, as is education of the family in the process of rehabilitation. It is the family who, in most instances, will be giving continued care in the community following discharge from the hospital.

Thoughts should be directed at a very early stage to the return to the community, and a home visit should be conducted as soon as practicable in order to provide stimulation for the patient, boost morale, and to assist in both short- and long-term planning. The initial home visit should not be seen as a way of emptying beds, but as a part of the treatment programme. An ill-planned and hurried discharge will result in a possible failed discharge and readmission.

A home visit should only be conducted when it is safe to do so, when the patient is medically stable and the family is strong enough to cope. Seeing the patient in his/her own home for the first time since injury will bring the consequences of the injury into reality and the family will need considerable support at this point in order to work through their expectations as compared to the reality.

Discharge should be planned and progressive, starting with short sessions at home, either escorted or unescorted, leading to overnight stays and trial leaves. Work will need to be done with the family and patient, both in the home and in the hospital, in order to ensure that necessary procedures can be carried out safely without injury to either patient or relative. Discharge from inpatient care should lead on to out-patient attendance for further rehabilitation.

Before discharge, patients should be provided with the relevant disability equipment and adaptations, as assessed for by skilled personnel from relevant agencies. Community services should be organized to commence on discharge if needed; if services are limited some activities may be continued in the hospital until the patient becomes independent or alternative support can be offered.

Headway, the UK's National Head Injury Association, has local branches in many parts of the country and the members provide support for both victims and relatives. It is important to introduce relatives to a group early on, and for staff to become involved as well.

Some patients will never improve sufficiently to return home, and these will need to be found long-term accommodation. The type of accommodation sought will depend on the amount of family involvement, possible compensation pending, and facilities within the area. Unfortunately, there is very little suitable accommodation for this group of patients.

There are also patients who have no home to go to, for whatever reason, and the team will need to assess the potential for recovery to independence in order to identify the future needs, and, therefore, plan for rehabilitation and care.

7

Psychosocial aspects

How often have those of us dealing with head-injured patients heard relatives say 'he's not the same person', 'he's not the man I married', 'he looks the same, but that's the only resemblance'. How difficult it is for any of us to put ourselves in their position and imagine what it is like to bring a stranger home instead of a well-loved husband, wife, son, daughter, mother or father. How difficult it is for us to imagine what it is like to have a loved one behaving in a manner most unlike anything seen before, remembering little of what she/he previously valued and being unable to carry out any of her/his past roles. We are told that empathy is more constructive than sympathy, but some circumstances stretch the imagination too far.

Of course not every case is as extreme as this and families manage to survive without too much stress. However, there are those who, understandably, are unable to cope with the traumatic change of circumstances and change in roles.

PERSONALITY CHANGE

Personality consists of a unique and complex collection of character-istics which combine to create a distinctive character. The patient's premorbid personality has an impact on recovery: strong-willed, self-motivated people who are driven to accomplish positive goals and demonstrate good track records tend to do better after injury than those who have shown psychological and emotional instability, with history of drug or alcohol abuse, poor work record and little motiva-tion (Adamovitch *et al.*, 1985).

It is not unusual, in the majority of cases, for the personality to change following head injury, either for the better, or, more often, for the worse. Personality traits, which appeared as minor characteristics, may, following head injury, become dominant. Certain characteristics may be masked by overwhelming tiredness, intolerance, irritability, aggressiveness and impatience or frustration. Symptoms of apathy or euphoria are also frequently seen.

Initially, personality change may be overlooked as the joy of seeing the patient survive, followed by rapid improvement over the first few weeks, fills the relatives with optimism and hope for a full recovery. The patient and relatives are in an unusual environment when together in hospital and distractions of hospital routine, treatment sessions and crowded wards detract from changes in personality; relatives seeing only what they want to see, or making excuses for changed behaviour or personality.

As an inpatient, and often following this, the focus of attention by patients and relatives (and often members of the multidisciplinary team) is on the physical symptoms presented. As an occupational therapist, I have often been frustrated by the obvious lack of importance placed on treatment of any disorder other than mobility, with many patients believing that all will be well when they can walk unaided. Yes, certainly the patient will be much more independent when she/he can walk unaided, but if one cannot remember where one is walking to, or has no friends to walk with because one's social skills are considerably reduced, or one cannot hold down a job because one cannot sustain attention or respond appropriately to authority, then mobility is really of very little value.

Once home, the changed personality gradually comes to light as the patient is seen in his/her own environment and comparisons can easily be made by those close to him/her. It is easy for relatives to expect greater things than the patient is able to give and when demands are not met, it can result in both parties experiencing anger and frustration making relationships even more difficult.

BEHAVIOUR

Undesirable behaviour can be learned in the hospital setting with some patients gaining attention by being disruptive, loud, or aggressive. Behavioural disorders are difficult to control in the general hospital setting because of the continuous change of care staff, the influences of visitors and being in an open ward.

For example, one patient adopted a tiger-like stance to staff of a ward, growling and scratching when people approached. Certain staff displayed fear to the patient, often running from the ward when confronted. Because of this response the patient often avoided doing purposeful activity and so the behaviour was positively reinforced. However, if a member of staff faced this patient with an assertive manner and expressed no fear he would comply with their wishes. Had the staffing of the ward been consistent so would the positive approach, and the undesirable behaviour may have stopped.

Because it was an open ward, this same man also interfered with other patients who would generally not challenge him because of the perceived outcome. The responses of other patients, or their visitors, cannot be controlled in general wards, making modification of behaviour difficult to achieve. For example, a patient on a female ward continually called out for a nurse, approximately 60 times over a five-minute period. The only time she was quiet was when eating, when being spoken to or when encouraged to quietly sing hymns with a nurse. In an effort to get a base-line, and to identify factors influencing this behaviour, the patient was unobtrusively observed for several sessions. It was found that the behaviour was being reinforced by several factors including the responses from the other patients who shouted back at the woman, starting with soothing noises gradually replaced with shouts of 'shut up'. One can hardly blame the other patients who could get very little rest or relaxation because of the continuous noise.

Initial phase

Initially, as the level of awareness improves and the patient starts to respond, there may be a conflict of interests. For example, if an aim of treatment is to encourage verbal communication, any speech is rewarded even if the first words consist of foul language. However, it is not desirable to continue to encourage only this type of language, so the emphasis must gradually change to reward appropriate speech only.

During this phase it is often difficult to encourage the relatives to reward only the desired behaviour for it will not have been long since the patient was in a life/death situation and the family will be very relieved that she/he is in the process of recovery. In this phase it is very easy to reward unwanted behaviour and this should be avoided. The process of early education of the family will, hopefully, help them to put the patient's behaviour into perspective.

In the initial phase, as already stated, we must look for causes of bizarre and meaningless behaviour or restless and aggressive acts, for these may be in response to difficulties in understanding or interpreting what she/he is experiencing. The team, including the relatives, must be consistent in dealing with unwanted behaviour while it lasts, for this may only be a transient phase. The psychologist should be consulted when behavioural problems are in evidence, no matter at what stage of recovery, and should be able to identify what is reinforcing this unwanted behaviour and how to deal with it effectively.

The patient needs to feel secure in his/her surroundings and will tend to test where the boundaries are for acceptable behaviour. Everyone dealing with the care of the patient must keep him/her within these boundaries by adopting a consistent approach, and by rewarding appropriate behaviour.

Modification of behaviour

Behaviour modification is a method of extinguishing unwanted behaviour, or of shaping existing behaviour into a more socially acceptable pattern. In order to identify where the problem lies, the behaviour must be broken down into component parts and dealt with individually by rewarding appropriate responses. When dealing with the problem one should initially define exactly what the problem is, when it is seen and identify any factors which may lead up to this behaviour.

The questions to be asked are:

1. What is the patient doing that is seen as a behavioural problem? Not what we *think* she/he is doing, but the actions seen.
2. Is this behaviour seen in all the settings to which she/he is exposed? Or is it seen only in one particular environment? If so, what is different about that environment, or in what the patient has to do there?
3. Is this behaviour consistent with all staff and visitors or is it confined to a few?
4. Is the behaviour seen regularly throughout the day and night, or more likely to be seen at specific times, for example first thing in the morning, always after a tiring event, during meal times?
5. Is there any identifiable event which precipitates this behaviour?
6. What is the chain of events when this behaviour is displayed? Is

the patient gaining some form of satisfaction from the action taken by others in response to his/her behaviour?

In order to identify the nature of the problem it may be necessary to observe the patient at frequent intervals, recording his/her behaviour and that of others around. What is recorded must be carefully structured in order to get a useful measure of the behaviour and to identify any significant factors which may be precipitating it. Once this information has been collated, a treatment approach should be planned and all staff informed of the action to be taken in response to the unwanted behaviour. Following a predetermined period of time, the patient should be observed again for a measurement of the unwanted behaviour, which will determine if the treatment has been effective and to what degree. This is a continuous process and the treatment approach should be regularly reviewed and modified as necessary.

It is recommended that a clinical psychologist is consulted before starting a behaviour modification programme because it can be very complex. The psychologist will, however, welcome specific information on the nature of the problem. It may be that the behaviour is as a result of frustration, perceptual disorders, confusion or pain and these will need to be ruled out.

Finding the correct reward for each patient for desired responses needs considerable thought and may include meaningful verbal praise, touch, cigarettes or sweets. The modification programme requires regular reviewing, particularly in the early days, for the patient should not become dependent on the reward. Rewards should always be immediate – if there is a delay the patient may forget what she/he is being rewarded for, or may be rewarded for undesirable behaviour displayed immediately before the giving of the reward.

It may be worth remembering that the tolerant and patient approach, adopted by many relatives during the weeks following injury, is not always a good thing as the patient may need to pick up intonation or non-verbal communication as a means of monitoring behaviour. For example, the wife of a patient writes:

'When he came home for the day this week we had our first argument (one thing I promised that we would never do again). He is now quite able to use a bottle but he just blankly refuses to to, so he pees wherever he happens to be. He did this in the first hour of being home, so I shouted at him that I was totally fed up with changing him and that he was being very selfish and just seeking attention.

His face dropped and he hung his head really low. However, it must have done the job because from that day he has never had an accident in the daytime again.'

Another woman, the mother of a 14-year-old head-injured patient, took her son home very early in his rehabilitation programme. He was at this time only able to swallow soft foods and was in the process of retraining in self-feeding. He was, however, uncooperative in this difficult activity, preferring to sit back and let other people do the work for him. On one occasion, his mother was encouraging him to feed himself a bowl of custard. As he became increasingly frustrated at not being fed by his mother, in anger he knocked the bowl away sending the contents spilling over his mother and the floor. His mother, also feeling extremely angry and frustrated, went into the kitchen for another bowl of custard, came back to her son and promptly poured the whole lot over his head. 'Did it work?' she was asked; he certainly didn't like it, was shocked but jolted into realizing just how wrong his behaviour had been.

I am not advocating the fighting of fire with fire (or custard with custard!), but patients need feedback on their behaviour and at an early stage this has to be in a basic form that they will understand. Relatives need also to be aware that reactions of frustration and anger are natural and should not always be controlled.

Aggression

This is not uncommon in our society and many situations call for an aggressive response; what we are referring to in this section is the inappropriate and often unprovoked use of aggression, either verbal or physical.

Aggression is not uncommon following head injury, but can be a transient phase which requires firm handling by all. This aggression may manifest itself as verbal or physical, or a mixture of both, and can be seen either as indiscriminate or triggered by a certain prompt.

If aggressive acts continue they will become a barrier to rehabilitation and therefore to a return to the community. The longer the aggression is reinforced the harder it will be to eventually modify. It will be reinforced by such acts as giving the patient continued attention during outbursts and displaying fear or anxiety when approaching him/her. If the patient is not expected to enter into therapeutic activity because of his/her aggressive behaviour, this will further reinforce it.

It should be of prime importance to prevent the patient from hurting him/herself or others; if mobile on an open ward, the other patients are as much at risk as the staff, and even the relatives and friends are subject to aggression (if not the prime objects). Restraining of the patient should be done with due consideration to the individual patient, taking advice where necessary from those experienced in restraining techniques. Staff attending the patient for restraining purposes may, however, reinforce this behaviour because she/he will be given attention unless dealt with quickly and quietly and removed to an area where there is no human contact. However, a quite place is difficult to find in most general hospitals. Where in an open ward can you carry out restraint of a patient without those with little understanding of its value believing that harm is being done? The team should, with the guidance of a psychologist, determine the approach to be adopted, taking into account the environment in which the patient is currently living; there may be no alternative placement for him within or outside the hospital. All staff should be aware of the adopted policies in the management of the potentially violent patient.

If the patient has a good relationship with a particular member of staff, she/he may be elected to deal with any crises that arise. She/he should be prepared to talk with the patient about the aggressive acts, but should not express dominance or aggression in return.

During the threat or act of violence, determine whether or not the situation can be diffused by approaches other than restraining ones, such as by using non-threatening, non-verbal stances, or soothing intonations to comfort and reassure the patient. If you feel that the patient is going to hit out, stand either very close or too far away to be an easy target. If the patient is being violent to either staff, patients or visitors, all staff should be prepared to assist. If you are the one being attacked, you must act responsibly in defending yourself. If the patient is violent against property, plan your action; saving furniture is not a priority.

Tying patients down in a bed or in a chair will generally increase frustration and agitation, and it is not to be recommended, particularly if alternatives are available. Sedating the patient achieves very little except temporary peace of mind for the other patients, visitors and staff.

If the patient is bored, she/he has the opportunity to dwell on her/his changed circumstances, and opportunities will arise which may encourage aggressive outbursts. A purposeful daily programme within occupational therapy and physiotherapy, as well as planned

119

ward-based leisure activities, may be all that is needed to divert the patient away from potentially explosive situations. Activities may also be planned which allow the patient to release aggression in a socially acceptable manner – for example throwing clay, bread-making, and active sports (the choice, of course, being according to the patient's level of function).

Consideration must be given to the feelings of the friends and family: it must be extremely alarming to see your loved one physically restrained, either by several people or by being tied down. They will need considerable support through this period. If an act of aggression occurs on the ward, staff involved should be given the opportunity to express their feelings, and colleagues should be available to offer their support.

Aggression may also continue into the long term and may be physically or verbally directed to immediate family or others close to the patient, or to property.

Apathy

The patient may become apathetic following injury and this also disrupts rehabilitation because of the difficulty in motivating him/her. There may be a tendency to withdraw from people or situations which cause considerable anxiety to the patient, for example from those situations which demand too much or are too difficult to cope with.

A patient may appear to be coping well when engaged in conversation on a superficial level and it may not be until she/he is forced into difficult activities or problem-solving situations that she/he becomes restless or irritable. If not receiving active rehabilitation, this may not be noticed until the patient is discharged and is expected to take on usual responsibilities within the home or at work.

Sexual behaviour

Sexual behaviour may be altered following head injury, with the patient experiencing either marked disinterest or increased drive. Early in recovery it is not unusual for the head-injured patient to masturbate anywhere and everywhere without inhibition. This is reinforced if the responses received are either those of laughter or expressions of horror, or if some other form of attention is drawn to it. This is most upsetting for relatives to witness. Masturbation should be dealt with quickly, firmly and without fuss, and if the patient is able to attend to conversation, time should be taken to explain the significance of his/her actions in public. If the patient continues to do this, on each occasion she/he should be taken immediately and without fuss to a quiet area, informed why, and left alone for a short period of time; this response should be a consistent one.

Hopefully this is just a phase that the patient goes through; generally it does not last. As the patient becomes more aware, it would serve no purpose to inform him/her of this past behaviour and it is best for all if it is forgotten.

The patient may also start to touch, or make other sexual advances to, members of the opposite sex and this again should be dealt with quickly and firmly without fuss. The behaviour should be discussed with the patient and it should be explained why it is undesirable.

Relatives may need help in understanding these actions, and, in the case of the spouse, may need help in coming to terms with their own possibly altered sexual feelings towards the patient, particularly if it is one of repulsion. The subject needs to be dealt with early in the rehabilitation process as situations are going to arise, particularly in home visiting, when partners will eventually be left alone together. It may be that, if not informed, relatives may be in doubt as to the advisability of sexual arousal in terms of health, or may be unsure if the sexual act will be possible. If this subject is presented by either the patient or the partner, if should be dealt with without embarrassment, and referred to a relevant agency, for example psychology, for appropriate counselling if you do not feel qualified to give sufficient help.

EFFECTS ON THE FAMILY

These consequences of head injury are of major concern and distress to the family and yet little is understood of the severity, nature and extent of the problems. It is only within the last 20 years that the burden that the head-injured patient places on the family and local community has been recognized. Patients were, and to a great extent still are, discharged on the ability of the family to cope with the physical aspects of injury, and much emphasis was (and unfortunately still is) placed on the progress of the patient within the physiotherapy department.

Evidence suggests, however, that physical disability on its own does not affect family cohesion. Rosenbaum and Najenson (1976), conducted a study in Israel comparing the wives of paraplegics and the wives of head-injured patients. They found that the wives of husbands who had suffered severe head injury were more likely to report drastic life changes, depressed mood, tense interpersonal relationships, loneliness and isolation and of having to assume the role of the husband. The head-injured person was commonly found to be dependent, childish, demanding and selfish.

In Glasgow, McKinlay et al. (1981), looked at the difficulties experienced by the head injured, as reported by their relatives, three, six and twelve months post injury. The number of physical problems reported initially were small and even smaller after one year. The most common problems reported at three months were those of slowness, tiredness and poor memory and at one year were those of irritability and impatience, as well as tiredness and poor memory.

A study by Brooks (1984), in which 134 head-injury patients were followed up over a period of five years, reported that the most common problems seen in this group (as reported by the relatives five years on) were those of irritability, anger, lability and being very demanding. Threats of violence were also commonly reported.

The effects on the family of a head-injured member returning home do not need to be spelt out if one considers the problems reported of irritability, tiredness, poor memory and impatience. Support is often forthcoming at the time of injury and the few months following, but as time goes on and progress appears to slow down, this is a time when the support from friends and distant relatives starts to drop off and the family members become increasingly isolated, lonely and depressed. This is the time when the other members of the family realize that their expectations have been unrealistically high, and they begin to understand what the future holds.

We can help the family, over the long term, by giving the relative(s) and the patient the opportunity to work through the inflicted changes. This may be done by any relevant professional, such as the psychologist, social worker or occupational therapist. The family will not be able to accept the new changed person unless they have the opportunity of mourning the loss of the old, and this is something that is difficult to do if the 'body' is still in the home. Local Headway meetings are a good forum for discussing the changes, as many members will have had similar experiences.

A big problem which often occurs following head injury is that of self-centredness, which is understandable as following injury the patient is a central focus of attention from relatives and friends. However, relatives have rights and needs as well, and as recovery occurs there may be gradual growth of resentment that the patient is so demanding, without, apparently, giving anything in return. Depression is commonly experienced by the patient where some insight is retained, if the patient is bitter about the outcome of the injury this may be taken out on those who care for his/her daily needs; the family members must be persuaded to look after their own mental and physical health in the long term without feeling guilty for putting their own needs before those of the head-injured family member.

In the home, the social life of the family unit may suffer because there are fewer opportunities to go out to meet friends, or friends may stop coming to visit because of even a minor change in personality, or a change in desire to follow certain leisure pursuits. Due to the demands made by the head-injured patient there may be less opportunity for individual family members to focus on each other's needs.

COGNITIVE IMPAIRMENT

Throughout the book it has been emphasized that one cannot work on one function at a time because of the high degree of interrelation. For example if perceptual disorders are present, the approach to physical disorders will have to take this into consideration, and if hearing is impaired communication will have to be through another intact sense.

Impairment of cognitive processes will have a significant effect on the patient's level of functioning and, therefore, on his/her level of independence – cognition being defined as the method the central nervous system uses to process information. Although it is the psychologists who will be the prime objective assessor of cognitive abilities, all team members will benefit from having knowledge of the relevant functions and alternative means of coping with disorders.

How the patient moves around and interacts with his/her environment under different work and social situations, and during performance in activities of daily living, will give an indication of the cognitive problems experienced. We may see a decreased level of attention, impaired memory, poor reasoning ability and reduced speed of information processing, as well as other problems.

Memory

Poor memory may be a problem following head injury and should be identified early on in the rehabilitation phase and strategies for coping should be adopted. It is a problem which should involve not only the rehabilitation team but also the whole family in its remediation as the patient may need to be given specific prompts, may rely on practice tasks, or may need to be encouraged to use aids such as diaries. The family will need to understand the problem in order to cope with its effects.

Poor memory will have an impact on rehabilitation because treatment programmes will have to take into account how much the patient can remember, what type of information she/he can cope with, and the span in which the information can be retained. In practical terms, she/he may not remember why it is necessary to carry out therapeutic activities, or that she/he has had an injury, and may not remember why she/he has to come to the hospital. All this does little for motivation.

The problems experienced by a head-injured person can be at any of the stages involved in remembering, that is, at the stage of initially correctly perceiving the information to be remembered; immediately holding the information; selecting how the information is to be stored; transferring the information into long-term memory; and retrieving the information when required. The psychologist should be able to identify where the process is breaking down and how best to cope with it.

The psychologist is not only concerned with assessment of where the deficit lies, but also with the extent of the functional problem, in identifying the best strategy for coping, and the approach to adopt in the rehabilitation programme. The problem should initially be defined, and this can be done by gathering information from the patient, from relatives, from therapists and through observation during activity.

Referral to a psychologist may be indicated if one or a combination of significant functional problems exist. These may include forgetting information within a short period of time, for example 10 minutes, even after prompting; experiencing difficulty remembering the names and faces of new people; forgetting how to get to places in the immediate environment; and frequently forgetting how to carry out specific activities.

Objective assessments are generally of very little value and will not give the interpreter information on how the patient performs. However, functional tests, such as the Rivermead Behavioural Memory Test, assess the patient's ability to remember names, routes, instructions, faces, stories and where things have been put; they measure the problem in practical terms.

Questionnaires may be useful in establishing the type of functional memory problem that the patient is experiencing and the ways of coping with it. The type of questions asked may include the patient's perceived level of ability to remember names of people, birthdays, faces, appointments, tunes or lyrics of a song, theme of a book or serial, jokes, giving messages, names of actors in films, and learning new skills and routes. Questions may include whether the patient has (and the perceived severity of) the following: problems of forgetting what he was going to do or say in the middle of doing or saying it, forgetting if one has locked the house or turned off the cooker etc., being unable to place faces or voices seen or heard before.

There may have been a memory problem prior to injury and this should be checked with the relatives. It is also important to know how the patient dealt with this problem, or, even if no problem existed, what methods the patient adopted premorbidly to remember information.

There is no evidence to suggest that practice on memory games, such as Kim's game, generalizes to improvement of memory in all aspects of function, although there may be an improvement in that practice task. The emphasis in treatment should be on compensating for this deficit by teaching appropriate strategies for coping. These strategies may include the use of a notebook or diary, use of lists, calendar or wall-chart, putting things to be remembered in an obvious place (external memory aids); teaching the patient to visualize or draw names to be remembered in picture form, or learning rhymes or stories made up to remember important information, and mental retracing of events (internal memory aids). It may be beneficial to change the environment in order to help the patient cope within it. This could be by means of signposting important areas such as the toilet, but the patient may also need practice in using these signs.

Problems exist in teaching the patient to cope with poor memory because she/he may not acknowledge that there is a problem, may not want to use external memory aids, may not remember to use external memory aids, and the patient's cognitive functioning may be such that it is difficult to teach the use of internal memory aids such as visual or first-letter mnemonics.

Living with someone who has a memory problem can be very stressful, particularly if it is so severe that independent living is no longer possible. Even if the problem is a minor or moderate one, the family may well have to keep repeating information, may have to repeatedly prompt the patient to complete tasks, and may have to cope with him/her forgetting to bring items of shopping home, forgetting where he/she is going and why, and forgetting to pass on messages or attend appointments. The patient him/herself may become very confused and agitated if his/her routine is interrupted and he/she cannot remember why. Every effort should be made to help the relative and the patient come to terms with this problem.

Attention

Following head injury the patient may experience difficulty in maintaining attention during the performance of a task at even the most basic level. Head-injury patients are generally orientated towards a stimulus and are therefore easily distracted. In a noisy or active area, the patient may experience difficulties in selecting the stimulus that they should be attending to and, once selected, difficulties may arise in maintaining attention.

It may be that a patient will function adequately and maintain attention during activity in a quiet, controlled area, or during social interaction. However, the same person can find it very difficult to attend to a task or conversation in a busy area, such as a workshop or a party. Thus, initially, rehabilitation should take place in a controlled environment, but recognizing the demands made on the individual in the community, the patient must be gradually introduced to greater distractions.

Poor attention will affect rehabilitation because the patient may not attend to instructions or may start to follow instructions when only half way through and therefore not fully understand the task in hand; if the task is not understood it has little meaning for the patient. The best way to assess attention is by observing the patient during activity and whilst following instructions.

During treatment, ensure that the patient has listened to the whole instruction before she/he starts the task and ask her/him to repeat if possible; this will slow the patient down and allow time for assimilating the information. During a session, be prepared to carry out several short activities rather than one long one, in order to maintain attention, starting with those which interest the patient.

At home, the family can be advised that it may be difficult for the patient to concentrate on a conversation if the television or radio is on, or if children are making a noise in or outside the room. If visitors call, they can be discouraged from holding several conversations in the same room so that the patient does not become confused and can concentrate on one person at a time.

It should also be remembered that what a patient could do automatically before his/her injury may take considerable concentration to perform afterwards. For example if mobility is a problem the patient may have to concentrate very hard on staying upright and will not therefore be able to attend to a conversation at the same time as walking. It may be difficult to attend to any two tasks at once and patients may have to stop what they are doing, either in therapy, or at home, to answer even a simple question.

Problem-solving

Following head injury, the patient may become very concrete in his/her thinking, lose the ability to analyse a problem, become very slow in thought-processing, and be unable to draw on past experience to solve a current problem.

In order to help a patient assimilate information, we must look at the rate at which she/he can take information in, the amount which she/he can cope with, the time during which she/he can attend to a task, the sense through which she/he is more able to understand information, and the degree of complexity that she/he is able to cope with (Barth and Boll, 1981).

After looking at these areas, we are able to identify where the patient is having difficulties and a treatment programme can be formulated in order to deal with these. The presentation of information can very gradually be, as the patient progresses, increased in its complexity at a rate which allows him/her to succeed.

The patient must first be encouraged to respond to his/her environment and to attend to the appropriate stimulation within it. When the patient starts to attend to the correct stimulation he/she has to be encouraged to organize and manipulate it correctly, and, following this, should be encouraged to formulate thoughts and ideas and utilize these in solving problems.

The difficulty in many hospital settings is that the patient is often not expected to think for him/herself or to make decisions. When he/she makes an error, correct feedback is not always given in order to help him/her adjust the performance next time and so the patient may not realize that a mistake has been made or where the error lies. Adequate feedback may not be given because it is easier to carry out tasks for the patient instead of encouraging him/her to do things independently, and many busy staff members who regularly handle the patient are neither aware of the need to provide feedback to the patient nor are they aware of what they should be looking for. Sometimes staff are only concerned with getting the patient from A to B. This leads to a masking of deficits which are not highlighted until the patient is put in a position where she/he is expected to be progressively independent in activities of daily living, and, in many instances, this may be when discharged.

SUMMARY

The effects of a severe head injury do not only last for a short period following injury but remain life-long problems which affect the injured person and the family. The patient cannot be treated in isolation from the family unit and relatives should be included in both the short- and the long-term treatment planning.

It is not uncommon to hear that patients have been discharged from hospital on the basis of physical progress with little consideration given to psychosocial consequences. With little support, it can be very difficult for families to survive the burden of looking after a head-injured person who bears little resemblance in personality or behaviour to the person who was loved, who is now unable to carry out any of his/her previous roles and who remembers little of what she/he previously valued and held dear.

In the hospital setting, efforts should be made to avoid encouraging poor behaviour. Throughout the treatment programme the patient should be encouraged to respond appropriately in behaviour to the situation and the relatives and staff should present a united approach regarding his/her behavioural management. It may be difficult for the family to be firm with the patient when in the initial phase of recovery because she/he will have been so near to the life/death situation, but education and support during this period will help them to understand how necessary this is. Even much later in the patient's management, it may be that some relatives are still unable to be firm, and this will cause problems in the long term.

If formal behaviour modification is necessary, the environment should be such that the rewards are easy to control. Within the general hospital setting it is very difficult to practise behaviour modification techniques because of the lack of an adequately controlled environment. However, if there is a behavioural problem which can be defined, the psychologist should be consulted and a strategy for remediation decided upon which must be adhered to by all staff and visitors. The strategy must be regularly reviewed.

One of the emphases of this book has been on the interrelation of all the functions of the human body. Impairment of cognitive processes have a significant effect on the patient's level of functioning and, therefore, the level of independence. All members of the treatment team should be aware of this so that the approach can be adapted accordingly in order to accommodate impaired memory, poor reasoning and reduced speed of information-processing. It is difficult to identify where the cognitive impairment lies, but it is important to determine this in order to help the patient process information.

If the patient within the hospital setting is not required to take part in a rehabilitation programme, and not encouraged to do things for him/herself, cognitive problems may be masked and will remain hidden until he/she returns home and attempts to resume normal living.

WHERE TO GO FROM HERE

Working with head-injured patients from the time of injury to discharge is only exposing the tip of an iceberg; one has only to go to any Headway meeting to realize that the problems are generally only just beginning when the patient is discharged.

Where do you go from here? With the great shortage of suitable rehabilitation facilities in the UK, treatment after discharge from hospital is very difficult to find so many patients are abandoned and the families are left to cope as best they can, with little support and with increasing isolation. Following head injury, if one is to reach the maximum level of recovery across the wide range of possible disorders, rehabilitation is likely to be needed over a long period of time. This needs to be away from the hospital environment where the sick role is encouraged; it is counterproductive to rehabilitation as it equates to passivity (Eames, 1987). The process of rehabilitation requires the active participation of the individual working towards independence.

Because the outcome, and therefore the needs, vary considerably from person to person, the structure of the rehabilitation service for head-injured patients needs to be wide ranging. The services required range from long-term care provision (for instance a nursing home) for those who are so severely impaired that they cannot be cared for in the community, through to sheltered workshops and educational programmes (Fussey and Giles, 1988). No such structure currently exists in the UK.

One cannot adequately stress the importance of training for all disciplines coming into contact with head-injured patients, in order to improve the efficiency of existing services and to raise awareness of the problems and their remediation or strategies for compensating. Similarly, further research is needed to improve the effectiveness of the rehabilitation services and to bring about greater understanding of the long-term needs.

It is up to all of us to continue to push for improved rehabilitation provision to meet the long-term needs of this continually expanding group of patients.

References

Abreu, B.C. and Toglia, J.P. (1987) Cognitive rehabilitation: a model for occupational therapy. *American Journal of Occupational Therapy*, **47**, 7, 439–48.

Adamovitch, B.B., Henderson, S. and Averbach, J.A. (1985) *Cognitive Rehabilitation of Closed Head Injured Patients: A Dynamic Approach* Taylor & Francis, London.

Ayres, A.J. (1979) *Sensory Integration and the Child*, Western Psychological Society, Los Angeles.

Baum, B. and Hall, M.K. (1981) Relationship between constructional paraxis and dressing in the head injured adult. *American Journal of Occupational Therapy*, **35**, 7, 438–42.

Bartholomaeus, E. (1975) An O.T. approach to the management of acute head injuries. *British Journal of Occupational Therapy*, Nov., 246–8.

Barth, J. and Boll, F. (1981) Rehabilitation and treatment of central nervous system dysfunction: a behavioural medicine perspective. *Medical Psychology: Contributions to Behavioural Medicine*. Edited by Propock, C. and Bradley, L. Academic Press, New York.

Bentley, S., Murphy, F. and Dudley, H. (1977) Perceived noise in a surgical ward, and on an intensive care area: an objective analysis. *British Medical Journal*, **2**, 1503.

Berrol, S. (1983) Medical assessment. *Rehabilitation of the Head Injured Adult*. Edited by Rosenthal, M., Griffith, E.R., Bond, M.R. and Millar, J.D. F.A. Davis Company, Philadelphia. Chap. 17, 231–8.

Bjornaes, H., Smith-Meyer, H., Valen, H., Kristensen, K. and Ursin, H. (1977) Plasticity and reactivity in unconscious patients. *Neuropsychologia*, **15**, 451–5.

Bobath, B. (1977) Treatment of adult hemiplegia. *Physiotherapy*, **83**, 310–13.

Brennon, J. (1959) Response to stretch of hypertonic muscle groups in hemiplegia. *British Medical Journal*, **1**, 1504–7.

Brooks, N. (Ed) (1984) *Closed Head Injury: Psychological, Social and Family Consequences*. Oxford University Press, Oxford.

Carr, J.H. and Shepherd, R. (1980) *Physiotherapy in Disorders of the Brain*. Heinemann, London.

Chew, S.L. (1986) Psychological reactions of intensive care patients. *Care of the Critically Ill*, **2**, 2, 62–5.

Chapman, C.E. and Wiesendanger, M. (1982) The physiological and anatomical basis of spasticity: a review. *Physiotherapy Canada*, **34**, 3, 125–36.

The Chessington O.T. Neurological Assessment Battery (COTNAB), Tyerman, R., Tyerman, A., Howard, P., Hadfield, C., (1986) Nottingham Rehab., 17 Ludlow Hill Road, West Bridgford, Nottingham NG2 6HD.

Concha, M.E. (1985) A review of apraxia. Paper presented at the Second European Congress of Occupational Therapy.

Cope, D.N. and Hall, K. (1982) Head injury rehabilitation: benefit of early intervention. *Archives of Physical Medicine and Rehabilitation*, **63**, 433–7.

Eames, P. (1987) Head injury rehabilitation: time for a new look. *Clinical Rehabilitation*, **1**, 53–7.

Eggars, O. (1983) *Occupational Therapy in the Treatment of Adult Hemiplegia*. William Heinemann Medical Books Ltd, London.

Farber S.D. (1982) *Neurorehabilitation: A Multisensory Approach*. W.B. Saunders, Philadelphia.

Foss, B.M. (Ed), (1966) *New Horizons in Psychology: 1*. Pelican, London.

Fussey, I. and Giles, G.M. (Ed), (1988) *Rehabilitation of the Severely Brain-Injured Adult: A Practical Approach*. Chapman and Hall, London.

Gordon, C. (1982) Practical approach to the loss of smell. *American Family Physician*, **26**, 192.

Graded Naming Test, McKenna P., Warrington, E., NFER-NELSON Publishing Company Ltd., Darville House, 2 Oxford Road East, Windsor, Berkshire SL4 1DF.

Groher, M. (1977) Language and memory disorders following closed head trauma. *Journal of Speech and Hearing Research*, **20**, 212–23.

Gruzzman, M. (1982) Reversal operation after brain damage. *Brain and Cognition*, **1**, 331–51.

Guidice, M.A. and Berchou, R.C. (1987) Post-traumatic epilepsy following head injury. *Brain Injury*, **1**, 1, 61–4.

Gulbrandsen, G.B., Kristenson, K. and Ursin, H. (1972) Response habituation in unconscious patients. *Neuropsychology*, **10**, 313–20.

Headway, National Head Injury Association, 200 Mansfield Road, Nottingham, NG1 3HX.

Jennett, B. (1983) Post traumatic epilepsy. Paper given at the International Conference on the Management of Traumatic Brain Injury, organized by Headway.

Jennett B. and Bond, B. (1975) Assessment of outcome after severe head injury. *Lancet*, **1**, 480.

Jennett, B., Teasdale, G., Galbraith, S., Braakman, R., Averzaat, C., Minderhoud, J., Heiden, J., Kurzet, T., Murray, G. and Parker, L. (1976) Prognosis of patients with severe head injury. *Acta Neurochirurugia Suppl.*, **28**, 149-52.

Jennett, B., Teasdale, G., Braakman, R., Minderhoud, J., Heiden, J. and Kurtze, T. (1979) Prognosis of patients with severe head injury. *Neurosurgery*, **4**, 4, 283–9.

Johnson, D.A. and Roethig-Johnston, K. (1988) Coma stimulation: a challenge to occupational therapy. *British Journal of Occupational Therapy*, **51**, 3, 88–90.

Johnston, M. (1984) *The Stroke Patient: Principles of Rehabilitation*. Churchill Livingstone, London. 2nd edn.

Kaplan, N. (1962) Effects of splinting. *Archives of Physical Medicine and Rehabilitation*, **43**, 565–9.

King, T.I. (1982) Plaster splinting as a means of reducing elbow flexor spasticity: a case study. *American Journal of Occupational Therapy*, **36**, 10, 671–3.

Keele, C.A., Neil, E. and Joels, N. (1982) *Samson Wright's Applied Physiology*. Oxford Medical Publications, Oxford. 13th edn.

LeMay, M. and Geschwind, N. (1978) Asymmetries of the human cerebral hemispheres. *Language Acquisition and Language Breakdown*. Edited by Carmazza, A. and Zuriff, E. Johns Hopkins University Press, Baltimore.

Lezak, M.D. (1983) *Neuropsychological Assessment*. Oxford University Press. New York. Rev. edn.

Mandelstam, D. (1977) *Incontinence*. Heinemann Health Books and the Disabled Living Foundation, London.

McKinlay, W.W., Brocks, D.N. and Bond, M.R. (1981) The short-term outcome of severe blunt head injury as reported by relatives of the injured person. *Journal of Neurology and Neurosurgical Psychology*, **44**, 527.

McPherson, J.J., Kreimeyer, D., Aalderks, M. and Gallagher, T. (1982) A comparison of dorsal and volar resting hand splints in the reduction of hypertonus. *American Journal of Occupational Therapy*, **36**, 10, 664–70.

Medical Disability Society, Working Party Report (1987) *The Management of Traumatic Brain Injury*. Published by The Development Trust for the Young Disabled.

Mill Hill Vocabulary Scale Synonyms Test, Raven J. *et. al*. NFER-NELSON Publishing Company Ltd., Darville House, 2 Oxford Road East, Windsor, Berkshire SL4 1DF.

National Adult Reading Test, Nelson H., NFER-NELSON Publishing Company Ltd., Darville House, 2 Oxford Road East, Windsor, Berkshire SL4 1DF.

Neuhaus, B.E., Ascher, E.R., Coullon, B.A., Donohue, M.V., Einbond, A., Glover, J.M., Goldberg, S.R. and Takai, V.L. (1981) A survey on rationales for and against hand splinting. *American Journal of Occupational Therapy*, **35**, 2, 83–90.

Ontario Society of Occupational Therapists Study Group on the Brain-Damaged Adult (1977) *Perceptual Evaluation Manual*.

Ottenbacher, K. (1980) Cerebral vascular accidents: some characteristics of occupational therapy evaluation forms. *American Journal of Occupational Therapy*, **34**, 368–71.

Pedretti, L. (1985) *Practice Skills for Physical Dysfunction*. Mosby, St Louis. 2nd edn.

Peterson, L.T. (1985) *Neurological Considerations in Splinting Spastic Extremities*. Produced by Rolyon Medical Products. Form 4-126.

Peterson, P., Goar, D. and Van Deusen, J. (1985) Performance of adults on the Southern California Visual Figure Ground Perception Test. *American Journal of Occupational Therapy*, **39**, 8, 525–30.

Rivermead Perceptual Assessment Battery, Whiting S., Lincoln N., Bhavani G., Cockburn J., (1985) NFER-NELSON Publishing Company Ltd., Darville House, 2 Oxford Road East, Windsor, Berkshire SL4 1DF.

Rosenbaum, M. and Najenson, T. (1976) Changes in life patterns and symptoms of low mood as reported by wives of severely brain-injured soldiers.

Journal of Consulting Clinical Psychology, **44**, 881.

Rosenthal, M., Griffith, E.R., Bond, M.R. and Millar, J.D. (Eds), (1983) *Rehabilitation of the Head Injured Adult*. F.A. Davis Company, Philadelphia.

Russell, W.R. (1932) Cerebral involvement in head injury. *Brain*, **55**, 549.

Sacks, O. (1985) *The Man who Mistook his Wife for a Hat*. Duckworth, London.

Siev, E. and Freishtat, B. (1976) *Perceptual Dysfunction in the Adult Stroke Patient: A Manual for Evaluation and Treatment*. Slack Inc., Thorofare, New Jersey, USA.

Southern California Figure-Ground Visual Perception Test, (1966) Ayres A.J., Western Psychological Services, Los Angeles.

Snook, J.H. (1979) Spasticity reducing splint. *American Journal of Occupational Therapy*, **33**, 10, 648–51.

Steed, A. (1986) Using the Steed cushion in the treatment of the flaccid hemiplegia. *British Journal of Occupational Therapy*, **49**, 2, 34–8.

Stratton, H. (1986) Keeping the patient in touch with reality. *Care of the Critically Ill*, **2**, 2, 22.

Sylvester, J. (1973) *Assessment of Perceptual Dysfunction in the Newly Brain-Damaged Adult*. Prince Henry Hospital, Sydney, New South Wales, Australia.

Tomlin, J. (1977) Psychological problems in intensive care. *British Medical Journal*, **2**, 441–3.

Trombly, C.A. and Scott, A.D. (1977) *Occupational Therapy for Physical Dysfunction*. Williams and Wilkins, Baltimore.

Turner, A. (1981) *The Practice of Occupational Therapy: An Introduction to Physical Dysfunction*. Churchill Livingstone, London.

Walsh, K.W. (1978) *Neuropsychology: A Clinical Approach*. Churchill Livingstone, London. 1st edn.

Walstrom, P.E. (1983) Occupational therapy evaluation. *Rehabilitation of the Head Injured Adult*. Edited by Rosenthal, M., Griffith, E.R., Bond, M.R. and Millar, J.D. F.A. Davis Company, Philadelphia. Chap. 19, 271–89.

Warner, J. (1983) *Helping the Handicapped Child with Early Feeding*. Winslow Press.

Warren, M. (1981) Relationship of constructional apraxia and body scheme disorders to dressing performance in adult CVA. *American Journal of Occupational Therapy*, **35**, 71, 432–7.

Weiffenbach, J.M. (1982) Variation in taste thresholds with human aging. *Journal of the American Medical Association*, **247**, 775.

Westerman, S.T. and Shrewsbury, N.J. (1981) 'How I do it' = Head and kneck. A targeted problem and its solution. *Laryngoscope*, **91**, 301–3.

Whiting, S. and Lincoln, N. (1980) An ADL assessment for stroke patients, *British Journal of Occupational Therapy*, **40**, 44–6.

Zoltan, BB. and Meeder Rykman, D. (1985) Head injury in adults. *Practice Skills in Physical Dysfunction*. Edited by Pedretti, L. Mosby. 2nd edn, Chap. 31, 436–61. St Louis.

Index